Handbook of Global Health, Security, and War

Handbook of Global Health, Security, and War

Edited by

Martin Bricknell

Professor of Conflict, Health and Military Medicine at
King's College London
London, United Kingdom

Richard Sullivan

Professor of Cancer & Global Health at
King's College London
London, United Kingdom

WILEY

This edition first published 2025

© 2025 John Wiley & Sons Ltd

The right of Martin Bricknell and Richard Sullivan to be identified as the authors of the editorial material in this work has been asserted in accordance with law.

Registered Offices
John Wiley & Sons, Inc., 111 River Street, Hoboken, NJ 07030, USA
John Wiley & Sons Ltd, New Era House, 8 Oldlands Way, Bognor Regis, West Sussex, PO22 9NQ, UK

For details of our global editorial offices, customer services, and more information about Wiley products visit us at www.wiley.com.

The manufacturer's authorized representative according to the EU General Product Safety Regulation is Wiley-VCH GmbH, Boschstr. 12, 69469 Weinheim, Germany, e-mail: Product_Safety@wiley.com.

Wiley also publishes its books in a variety of electronic formats and by print-on-demand. Some content that appears in standard print versions of this book may not be available in other formats.

Library of Congress Cataloging-in-Publication Data applied for:
Paperback ISBN: 9781394326099

Cover Design: Wiley
Cover Images: © CDC (Centers for Disease Control and Prevention)/Wikimedia commons, © Boris Niehaus/Wikimedia commons, © National Archives/Wikimedia commons, © Nenea hartia/Wikimedia commons, © Imperial War Museums/Wikimedia commons, 'And the Band Played On' 2015 by Eleanor Crook, © the artist and Gordon Museum - KCL

Set in 10.5/13pt STIXTwoText by Straive, Pondicherry, India

Contents

Author Biographies

Dr Kiran Attridge, MBBS, MSc, MRCGP, FFPH, DMCC
Kiran Attridge is a Public Health Physician and GP. She completed her undergraduate medical studies at the University of Newcastle Upon Tyne and her postgraduate degree at the London School of Hygiene and Tropical Medicine. She saw first-hand the impact of war on health during her military service with the Royal Air Force, serving in Afghanistan and the broader Middle East before commencing her speciality public health training, where she focused on large-scale outbreak response in resource-poor and humanitarian settings, including DRC, Pakistan, and Sierra Leone. She is currently the Course Director for the Conflict and Catastrophe Medicine Course at the Centre for Health Studies at the Worshipful Society of the Apothecaries.

Ana Elisa Barbar
Ana Barbar is an expert on protection of healthcare, with a focus on safe health responses, civil-military relations and ethical challenges for provision of care in emergency settings. Ana Elisa currently works as a consultant to the World Health Organization and other humanitarian organizations. Previously, she worked for almost a decade in the Red Cross and Red Crescent Movement in different roles, working in Latin America, Middle East, and Africa and spent four years as global advisor to health policy and operations of the International Committee of the Red Cross on issues of protection of healthcare. Ana Elisa is the chair of the board of Insecurity Insight, and holds a Bachelor's in Psychology, with a clinical license and a full residency in Primary Health Care, as well as an Executive Master's in Policy Making and International Negotiations. As a guest lecturer, she has taught in different universities in Europe and Africa and served as an expert on protection of healthcare to high-level panels, including at the Economic and Social Council of the United Nations and to the Human Rights Committee of the National Academies of Sciences, Engineering, and Medicine of the United States. Her most recent publications include an article for *Daedalus* and a co-edited book on Medical Neutrality.

Dr Gemma Bowsher, BSc, MA, MBBS, FRSPH, FRGS
Gemma Bowsher is a physician-social scientist based at King's College London. She completed her medical degree at King's College London and her master's degree at Harvard University. She holds fellowships of the Royal Society of Public Health and the Royal Geographical Society. Her work spans operational and policy domains relating to health security threats in conflict settings such as Ukraine and the Middle East. She leads a range of programmes in these settings focused on responding to biological and chemical emergencies at the clinical, technical, and policy levels.

Jessica Bricknell, MMath, MSc (Associate Editor)

Jessica Bricknell has a master's in mathematics from the University of Nottingham, a master's in International Development from the University of Edinburgh and is an ACA chartered accountant. She has been working for the past eight years in the humanitarian and development sector, including the last five years across Uganda and South Sudan working for Save the Children.

Lieutenant General (Rtd) Professor Martin Bricknell, CB, OStJ, PhD, DM, FFPHM, FIHM

Martin Bricknell started as Professor of Conflict, Health, and Military Medicine at King's College London in 2019. Previously, he served 34 years in the UK Defence Medical Services, culminating his service as the Surgeon General of the UK Armed Forces. He undertook operational tours in Afghanistan, Iraq, and the Balkans with numerous additional overseas assignments. In 2010 and 2006, he held senior Medical Adviser appointments in the NATO ISAF mission. He was awarded the Companion of the Order of Bath, the Order of St John, and the US Bronze Star. He is a specialist in General Practice, Public Health and Occupational Medicine. His multiple academic papers cover: how organisations learn, care pathways in military healthcare, military healthcare ethics, civil-military relations in health, and the political economy of health in conflict. He convenes an MA module in Global Health, Security and War, and co-convenes an MA module in Conflict and Health. He is also Co-Director of the KCL Centre for Conflict and Health Security, the KCL Centre for Military Ethics, Veterans Adviser for the King Edward VII Hospital, Editor-in-Chief of the Military Medical Corps Worldwide Almanac, a non-resident Fellow of the Centre for Global Development, and on the editorial board for the *Journal of Military and Veterans Health*.

Dr George Bundy, MD (Associate Editor)

George Bundy is a PhD candidate based in the Department of War Studies at King's College London, where he researches Security Sector Health Systems in NATO Eastern Flank countries. After earning his medical degree from St. Petersburg State Pavlov Medical University, he completed a postdoctoral fellowship at the University of Toledo College of Medicine. His work spans clinical practice, biomedical, and public health research, addressing global health security threats and strengthening health systems across multiple countries.

Dr Eddie Chaloner, BA(Oxon), BM, BCh, FRCS, Gen

Eddie Chaloner is a recently retired vascular surgeon. He served in the British Army and also worked in a variety of conflict/post-conflict settings with NGOs, including the HALO Trust and Medicins Sans Frontiers. He has published widely on the treatment of blast injury, particularly from anti-personnel landmines. His current interest encompasses the study of war more generally in its socio-political context, particularly in relation to the emerging field of cognitive warfare.

Professor Peter von Dadelszen, DPhil (Oxon), FRANZCOG, FRCSC, FRCOG

Peter von Dadelszen is Professor of Global Women's Health and Honorary Consultant Obstetrician. He is an obstetrician-scientist at King's College London and King's

Health Partners. A New Zealander (and now Canadian), Peter trained clinically and academically in New Zealand, UK, and Canada. Currently, his research focus is on pregnancy hypertension, fetal growth, preterm birth, and stillbirth, through a One Health lens.

Colonel (Rtd) Dr Sohrab Dalal, MSc, MSc, MRCGP

Sohrab Dalal trained in medicine at Guy's Hospital Medical School in the 1980s and completed postgraduate training in primary care in London. Working part-time in the Faculty of Primary Care at King's College, London, and as a GP in London, he developed an interest in medical education. Dr Dalal spent three decades working for the UK Ministry of Defence, gaining experience in Aviation Medicine, combat casualty care and Emergency Medicine. Dr Dalal deployed over this period to the broader Middle East Region, including Iraq, Afghanistan, and Syria with UK, coalition and other nation's forces, for which he was awarded the Meritorious Service Medal. Dr Dalal was appointed a postgraduate trainer and holds master's degrees in International Primary Care and Defence Leadership. More recently, he held the positions of Regional Clinical Director (North England) and Head, Medical Branch at NATO HQ Supreme Allied Command Transformation (2018–2022), where he was responsible for the creation of the NATO Medical Support Capstone Concept and Allied Joint Publication 4.10c, *Medical Support to Operations.*

Dr Catherine Davison, MBChB, MA, MRCGP (Associate Editor)

Catherine Davison is a highly experienced senior medical leader with a 21-year career in the Royal Air Force (RAF). A trained General Practitioner, she has worked extensively in global remote and challenging environments, holding key roles in operational planning, policy development, and medical leadership across diverse international settings. As Commander of the Tactical Medical Wing, she led a 160-member unit capable of deploying medical capabilities worldwide at high readiness. Her recent experience includes overseeing medical support for NATO and the United Nations, managing a NATO Role 2 facility, and leading United Nations Medical Assistance Teams (MATs) and Aero-Medical Evacuation Teams (AMETs). Catherine also served as Deputy Force Medical Officer for the United Nations Mission in South Sudan (UNMISS), where she was responsible for healthcare delivery in support of peacekeeping operations. Her career has focused on planning and implementing medical support for international missions, crisis response, and providing care in austere environments.

Dr Abdulkarim Ekzayez, MD, PhD

Abdulkarim Ekzayez is a health system expert with over 13 years' experience in clinical medicine, humanitarian health, epidemiology, health in conflict settings, and academic research. With in-depth knowledge of the principles as well as the practicalities of health interventions and dynamics in conflict settings, he has a proven ability in developing strategies, operational plans, research, and evidence-based policies for health interventions in contested conflict settings. His key achievements include: building one of the first primary health care systems in northwest Syria, which included the development of locally customised electronic medical records; leading the Polio vaccination response in northern Syria between 2013 and 2016; developing an evidence-based strategy for the Ministry of Health in Afghanistan to introduce new medical interventions in 2018; leading a global research project on reporting attacks on healthcare in conflict settings with the Chatham House in 2019; designing and co-leading the Research for Health Systems Strengthening in northern Syria (R4HSSS) project, a large multidisciplinary operational research project on health system strengthening in Syria led by King's College London.

Dr Rachael Gribble, PhD, MSc

Rachael Gribble is a Lecturer in War and Psychiatry at King's College London, UK. As a mixed methods researcher with a background in public health, the primary focus of her work is on how occupation influences the well-being of families. To date, her work with military families has included spouse/partner employment, family separation, intimate partner violence, spouse/partner health and well-being, relationship satisfaction, adolescent health and wellbeing within military families, reservist families, partner identity, parents of veterans, and the experiences of LGBT+ personnel and veterans.

Dr Zenobia Homan, PhD

Zenobia Homan coordinates international professional development courses, workshops and related capacity building on chemical, biological nuclear and radiological (CBRN) security at the Centre for Science & Security Studies (CSSS) and King's Institute of Applied Security Studies (KIASS) of King's College London. She currently conducts research relating to security culture, education, communication and access to information with a focus on the development of exercises, case studies and multilingual methodologies. In the context of global health and conflict, she has worked on civil-military cooperation, One Health in complex settings, and resilience to chemical attacks. Dr Homan holds a BA Joint Honours degree from Durham University, MPhil from the University of Cambridge, and PhD from SOAS, University of London.

Colonel (Rtd) Professor David Ross, OStJ, PhD, MSc, FRCPCH, FFPH, FFTM, FRCP

David Ross retired from the Royal Army Medical Corps after 41 years' service. He led the Defence Public Health cadre for 15 years. David was appointed the Parkes Professor of Preventive Medicine in 2012, an Honorary Queen's Physician in 2014 and an Officer in the Order of St John in 2023. His professional interests have focused on Health Protection, Humanitarian Medicine, Travel Medicine, Infectious Diseases, Child Public Health, and Medical Education. David is Dean at the Worshipful Society of Apothecaries and was the Chief Examiner of the Diploma of Medicine in Conflict and Catastrophes from 2019 to 2023; Dean at the Faculty of Travel Medicine, Royal College of Physicians and Surgeons, Glasgow; and Chief Examiner for the Final MFPH at the UK Faculty of Public Health. He led a mixed methods research project into risk factors for mental ill health in the Army and was awarded a PhD for this work from the University of Glasgow in 2024.

Dr Lucy Singh, MSc (Dist), MBChB, BSc, MMedSci (Hons)
Lucy Singh is an NIHR Academic Clinical Fellow in Obstetrics and Gynaecology at King's College London. She completed her medical degree at the University of Aberdeen and her MSc Reproductive and Sexual Health Research with distinction at the London School of Hygiene and Tropical Medicine. Her work currently focuses on maternal near-miss events in low-resource and conflict-affected settings.

Air Vice-Marshal (Retd) Professor Tracy Smart, AO, MPH, MA, FRACMA, FACAsM, FAsMA, FCDSS, FACHSM (Hons)
Tracy Smart is a doctor, aerospace medicine specialist, and retired Royal Australian Air Force senior officer. During 35 years of service, she deployed to Rwanda, Timor Leste, the Middle East and Lebanon and undertook leadership and command positions at all levels. She was Surgeon General of the Australian Defence Force and Commander Joint Health from 2015 to 2019. Professor Smart's current roles include Professor of Military and Aerospace Medicine at the Australian National University, Director of Goodwin Aged Care and the Australian College of Aerospace Medicine, member of the Defence Honours and Awards Appeals Tribunal, and co-chair of the Australian War Memorial Redevelopment Project's Veterans' Advisory Group.

Professor Richard Sullivan, MD, PhD
Richard Sullivan is Professor of Cancer and Global Health at King's College London. He is the Director of the Institute of Cancer Policy and the Centre for Conflict and Health Security. Richard is a NCD advisor to the World Health Organisation and a Fellow at the Centre for Global Development. He has led several major research programs in conflict and health with a special interest in the Middle East and cancer control in conflict settings. He trained in surgical oncology with a PhD in Biochemistry from University College London. Richard was previously Clinical Director of Cancer Research UK and past Director of the Council for Emerging National Security Affairs.

Dr Adarsh Tiwathia, MBBS, MS, CIME
Dr Adarsh Tiwathia retired from the role of the Deputy Director of the Division of Healthcare Management and Occupational Safety and Health of the United Nations in 2025. In this role, she oversaw the health, safety and well-being of all UN personnel deployed around the globe. Her responsibilities included delivering a standardized and quality healthcare system along with Public Health and Occupational Health to all UN personnel worldwide.

She has provided leadership on healthcare management to over 150 UN healthcare facilities and has worked to set global standards on the various aspects of delivery of healthcare to UN personnel. She has designed and implemented a UN-wide accountability framework for healthcare services, which includes a system for ensuring adherence to UN Healthcare Quality and Patient Safety Standards; a system for continuous improvement of services through conducting Root Cause Analysis and patient experience surveys; and an environment in which clinical excellence flourishes by promulgating clinical pathways and conducting clinical audits to ensure compliance. Dr Tiwathia has engaged in building Health Systems in field settings, especially in conflict areas. Before joining the United Nations, Dr Tiwathia served in the Indian

Army Medical Corps at the UN Dispensary in Hanoi, Vietnam; and worked with NGOs engaged in Public Health Programs including HIV/AIDS.

Ben Wakefield, MSc, DIntS, FRGS

Benjamin Wakefield is a British international security expert focused on biological security, global health security and broader CBRN issues. His work aims to better understand, develop, and improve emergency preparedness for natural, accidental, and deliberate biological events. He is currently a Specialist Senior Advisor in the UK Government Cabinet Office's National Security Secretariat. Previously, he was a Senior Analyst at the Johns Hopkins Center for Health Security, the Deputy Director of the Center's Emerging Leaders in Biosecurity Initiative (ELBI) Fellowship Program, and held several roles at the Royal Institute of International Affairs (Chatham House). He was also a consultant for the Stockholm International Peace Research Institute (SIPRI), a 2020 OSCE–UNODA Peace and Security Scholar and a 2020/2021 ELBI Fellow. Ben is a Fellow of the Royal Geographical Society and an alumnus of University College London, Loughborough University, and the University of Technology Sydney.

Dr Geoff Whitman, PhD

Geoff Whitman is a Lecturer in Global Health Education at King's College London. He is an Interdisciplinary Social Scientist. His research focuses on the relationships between knowledge, expertise, government policy, and the public, covering topics such as climate change, flooding, pollution, and urban green infrastructure. He also uses experimental participatory approaches to find ways of increasing public involvement in both the issues and solutions to problems that impact them, particularly in developing research that promotes the co-production of knowledge. Geoff has integrated these research interests into his lecturing and leads the Global Burden of Disease and the Conflict and Health modules, as well as the Introduction to Global Health for second year medical students on the MSc in Global Health at King's. Dr Whitman is currently developing a module on Climate Change and Health for both the MSc in Global Health and the MSc in Public Health.

Preface 1

The Charter of the United Nations is looking increasingly fragile, originating as it did as the global settlement for relations between sovereign states following the Second World War. The contemporary context reveals levels of violence between states in Eastern Europe and the Middle East that are approaching those experienced in the World Wars of the twentieth century; violence within civil wars in Africa and Asia that is driving substantial human migration; and an existential threat of conflict flaring in the South China Sea, with as yet unrealised consequences for global health and human security.

Yet war is a predictable and inevitable outcome when politics fails, as states strive to ensure their national security and protect their national interests. War of course inflicts a substantial cost on human security – either directly through death and injury, or indirectly through damage to health systems. This results in excess all-cause mortality and undermines the key determinants of health. Beyond conflict and war, the COVID-19 pandemic has been a reminder that health threats *per se* can independently impact the wider dimensions of global and national security in the economic, diplomatic and information domains – the latter relating to cyberattack and disinformation.

This book is timely for understanding an increasingly unstable world and the organisation of the response to crises that affect the health of populations. The co-editors have convened an impressive array of collaborating authors, bringing together a work that unifies concepts from security studies and biomedical studies in an accessible form for students and practitioners from both the humanities and the health sciences.

Unintentionally, but reassuringly, this mirrors my own professional career from a provider of emergency medicine to strategic leadership of the military medical services of NATO. It is a journey that has taken me from acute clinical practice; through public health and occupational medicine; to international relations, strategic studies, and practical aspects of health diplomacy on an international stage. I commend this book as an interdisciplinary primer that signposts the reader to additional resources that will support learning in global health, security, and war. I truly wish I had been afforded access to such a book 30 years ago as I embarked on my own journey to improve patient outcomes at the health systems level in peace, disaster, conflict, and war.

Timothy Hodgetts, CB, CBE, KHS, DL, DSc (Hons), PhD, MMEd, MBA
Major General (Rtd) Professor
Former Chairman of the NATO Committee of Chiefs of Military Medical Services
Former Surgeon General of the UK Defence Medical Services
Author of *Frontlines and Lifelines: Collected Poems from an Army Doctor in Crisis and War*. Unicorn Publishing, 2024.

Preface 2

Threats to health can be threats to national security. Conflict and wars have a direct impact on the health of affected populations, and health systems and services. These affect the resilience of societies to absorb and respond to external aggression. The COVID-19 crisis demonstrated the direct impact of a health crisis on non-health determinants of national security such as economic activity, financial stability, education, and societal cohesion. Senior health practitioners need to understand how their role in global health is informed by non-biomedical topics such as international relations, security studies, international development, International Humanitarian Law, and healthcare ethics in crises. These topics are not normally covered in books and courses on global health yet are an essential part of the knowledge base needed by health practitioners who work in complex security environments. The chapters in Part 1 of this book address this gap.

War is a catalyst for innovation in preventive medicine, pre-hospital care, hospital care, and rehabilitation for the injured, both physically and mentally. My professional career has been driven by my experiences of leading and managing military health services in conflict and peace. This has required a system-level understanding of civilian and military health systems at both a national and international level. I have also needed to understand the core clinical principles of trauma care, communicable disease, maternal and child care, non-communicable disease, and mental health care. Part 2 provides an excellent summary of these dimensions of a health system response to complex emergencies. These chapters provide the baseline knowledge needed by non-clinicians and signposts to deeper knowledge for health professionals.

The final part of this book provides insights into the processes of generating evidence and influencing policymakers to support strategic change. My senior career has been underpinned by the use of research to inform my own decisions and to advocate for organisational and political change. This part also provides signposts for early career professionals to develop their own skills to undertake research that is safe and ethical, and to develop their own careers.

Overall, this book is a fantastic aggregation of multi-disciplinary knowledge from highly respected experts. I believe that it is an essential guide for practitioners in the fields of global health, security, and war.

David Smith
Rear Admiral (Rtd)
Deputy Assistant Secretary of Defense for
Health Readiness Policy and Oversight
US Department of Defense

Abbreviations

Abbreviation	Meaning
ABC	airway, breathing, circulation
6Ps	prior planning prevents problems and poor performance
ABCDE	airway, breathing, circulation, disability, exposure
AI	artificial intelligence
AMR	antimicrobial resistance
ARS	acute radiation syndrome
BEmONC	Basic Emergency Obstetric and Newborn Care
BW	biological weapons
CBRN	chemical, biological, radiological, nuclear
CBT	cognitive behavioural therapy
CONSORT	Consolidated Standards of Reporting Trials
COPD	chronic obstructive pulmonary disease
COVID	coronavirus disease
CPMS	Child Protection Minimum Standards
CRSV	conflict-related sexual violence
CSCATTT	command and control, safety, communications, assessment, triage, treatment, transport
CW	chemical weapons
DCR	damage control resuscitation
DCS	damage control surgery
DDR	disarmament, demobolisation, reintegration
DIME	diplomatic, information, military, economic
EDRM	(health) Emergency and Disaster Risk Management
EmONC	Emergency Obstetrics and Neonatal Care
EMT	emergency medical team
EP Hum	package of essential palliative care for humanitarian emergencies and crises
EPPRR	emergency prevention, preparedness, response, and resilience
EQUATOR Network	Enhancing the Quality and Transparency of health Research Network
ERW	explosive remnants of war
FCAS	fragile and conflict affected situations
FPV	first-person view (drones)
GCs	Geneva Conventions
GHS	global health security

GHSA	Global Health Security Agenda
GHSI	Global Health Security Initiative
GHSI	Global Health Security Index
HIC	high-income country
IA	international agency
IDP	internally displaced person
ICMI	integrated management of childhood illness
ICRC	International Committee of the Red Cross
IHL	international humanitarian law
IHR	International Health Regulations
iNGO	international non-government organisation
IOM	International Organisation for Migration
JEE	joint external evaluation (of IHR 2005 capabilities)
LMIC	low and middle income (countries)
LOAC	laws of armed conflict
MARCH	massive bleeding, airway, breathing, circulation, heat (prevent and treat hot and cold injuries)
MDG	millennium development goal
MHE	military healthcare ethics
mhGAP-HIG	mhGAP humanitarian intervention guide
MHP	military healthcare practitioner
MHPSS	mental health and psychosocial support
MIDFIELD	military, information, diplomatic, financial, intelligence, economic, legal, and development
MIMMS	major incident medical management and support
MIRA	Multi-cluster/sector Initial Rapid Needs Assessment
MISP	minimum initial service package for sexual and reproductive health in crisis situations
NATO	North Atlantic Treaty Organisation
NCD	non-communicable disease
NGO	non-government organisation
NSAG	non-state armed group
PEN	package of essential noncommunicable disease interventions for primary healthcare
PEN-H	package of essential noncommunicable diseases interventions for humanitarian settings
PFA	psychological first aid
PHEIC	public health event of international concern
PRISMA	preferred reporting items for systematic reviews and meta-analysis
PTE	potentially traumatic event
PTSD	post-traumatic stress disorder
RoL	Rule of Law
SASE	safe and secure environment
SDG	sustainable development goal
SGBV	sexual and gender-based violence
SRH	sexual and reproductive health

SSR	security sector reform
STANAGS	NATO Standardisation Agreement
STI	sexually transmitted infection
UHC	universal health coverage
UN	United Nations
UN OCHA	United Nations Office for the Coordination of Humanitarian Affairs
UNGA	United Nations General Assembly
UNSC	United Nations Security Council
VPD	vaccine-preventable diseases
WASH	water, sanitation, and hygiene
WHA	World Health Assembly
WHO	World Health Organization
WPS	women in peace and security

Introduction

The 21st century has seen an unprecedented range of threats to health that have had a global impact on the security of populations, states, and the global system. The COVID-19 pandemic has been the most dramatic manifestation of the impact of a health crisis on health, economic stability, and global security. However, this is just one of many global crises with a substantial effect on the health of affected populations. Other infectious diseases have had pronounced effects on human and animal health and security, include severe acute respiratory syndrome (SARS), Middle East respiratory syndrome (MERS), Ebola, and foot-and-mouth disease.[1] Interstate and intrastate conflict has killed, injured, and disrupted health systems in the Middle East, South America, Africa, Asia, and Europe. Climate change is forecasted to further destabilise communities, leading to even greater human migration and health challenges across migration routes. The aim of this book is to introduce the inter-relationships between health, security, and war in order to place these in context for students studying global health, security, war, peace, humanitarianism, and development. The book is designed to support the reader's exploration of these topics either as a primer for self-directed learning or to complement formal education.

The book title has been chosen to engage the reader with the multiple dimensions of the relationships between security and health. It is set from a global perspective, whilst acknowledging the referent perspectives of national security and human security. Thus, this book covers much more than just the narrow definition of "global health security" as a public health response to threats from infectious diseases. By extension, it also examines the health consequences of the ultimate form of insecurity, war. Figure I.1 illustrates this approach.

The book introduces the academic theories underpinning each of these topics and then examines the impacts of insecurity and war on health systems, clinical health services, and the research and policy agendas. After this introduction, the first part covers different perspectives on health and security. Chapter 1 defines global health and the relationships between determinants of health, health systems, and health services. Chapter 2 discusses security from the three dimensions of human security, state security, and global security, and their relationships with health. Chapter 3 analyses the health impacts of the worst forms of insecurity, conflict, and war. Chapter 4 examines the new topics in globalisation of climate change and human migration as threats to the health of vulnerable populations. Chapter 5 summarises military technologies, how they are designed to kill and maim, and the biomedical sciences of treatment. Chapter 6 outlines international humanitarian law and ethics as constraints on the worst excesses of war and human barbarism. Chapter 7, the final chapter in this part, looks at the meaning and interpretation of the term "global health security" and its function in placing health within security agendas.

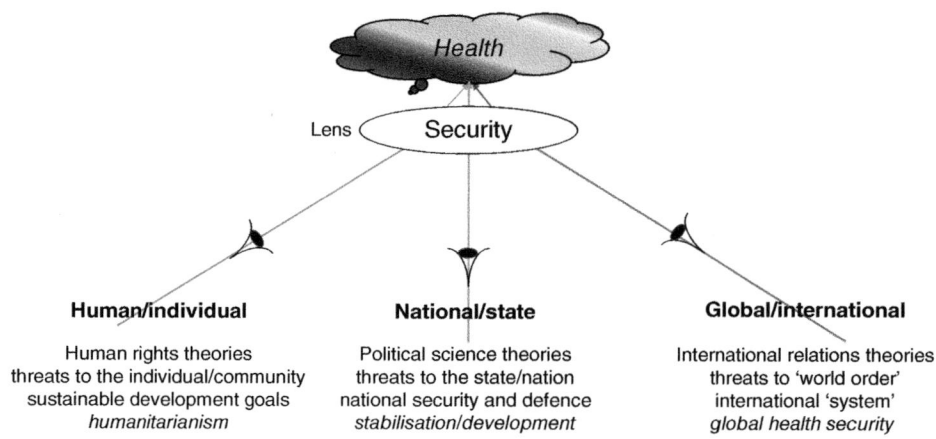

FIGURE I.1   Perspectives on health and security.

The chapters in Part 2 are more clinically orientated and consider the dimensions of a health service response to insecurity and war. Chapter 8 builds upon the concepts introduced in Chapters 1 and 3 by looking at the roles of national and international health systems in the response to crises and war. The subsequent chapters cover physical trauma (Chapter 9), communicable disease (Chapter 10), child health and sexual and reproductive health (Chapter 11), non-communicable disease and palliative care (Chapter 12), and lastly mental health (Chapter 13).

The final part integrates the previous two parts and examines the research and policy implications of globalisation, health, security, science, and war. Chapter 14 looks at how the research agenda needs to use multi-disciplinary and inter-disciplinary approaches to understand the causes and impact of insecurity and war on health, including providing a voice for vulnerable and marginalised populations. Chapter 15, linking to Chapter 2, discusses the development of security policies and the applications of the dimensions of national power in support of national and international security. It will show how health threats and the health consequences of insecurity and war have become more prominent in the security discourse. The final chapter (Chapter 16) concludes the book and provides readers with a guide and markers toward the future of these topics.

The chapters of the book have been designed to provide a handrail that enables readers to access and interpret the large volume of academic literature, policy papers, and clinical guidelines relevant to practice in global health, security, and war. Each chapter opens with a short introduction to the topic. It then sets out the learning objectives that determine the structure of chapter. A short self-study exercise frames the topic for the reader. The main body of the chapter covers the core dimensions of the topic and culminates in a case study or other example of the concepts of the chapter in practice. Each chapter is supported by a reference list of multimedia key sources of information including authoritative websites, policy documents, salient academic publications, and suitable videos or other media. This style enables readers to find new or contemporary information that will augment the material presented in this handbook.

The overall learning outcomes from studying this book are to:

- Set the foundations for a systematic understanding of interdependent concepts from the fields of global health, international relations, and security studies, as they relate to the analysis of global health, security, and war.
- Familiarise readers with foundational concepts underlying health threats as risks to human, national, and global security.
- Explore the role of health sciences and health services in the development of national and supra-national capabilities to protect healthcare services and other critical national security infrastructures.
- Provide frameworks for the original analysis of the historical and contemporary role of health sciences in the advancement of strategic objectives driven by security agendas.
- Foster critical analysis of the first-, second-, and third-order impacts of insecurity and conflict on health, and vice versa.
- Understand the key components of the clinical services that are needed to meet the health needs of populations affected by insecurity and conflict.
- Interpret the implications of a range of case studies of health crises on human, national, and global security by reference to historical examples and contemporary analysis.

This book is structured to align with the Sphere Handbook. This handbook is one of the most widely known and internationally recognised tools for humanitarian response. It comprises the Humanitarian Charter, the Protection Principles, the Core Humanitarian Standard, and minimum humanitarian standards in four vital areas of response: water supply, sanitation, and hygiene (WASH) promotion; food security and nutrition; shelter and settlement; and health [1]. This book is mainly concerned with the health response.

The content has been built around the editors' collective experience of teaching these topics at master's and PhD levels to students of global health, health security, international relations, and security studies. Our collective goal has been to make this subject accessible to practitioners across these academic disciplines. The authors have considerable practical experience in this field that underpins their academic credibility as researchers and teachers. We would like to thank our co-authors for the insights and experience that they have brought to their chapters. We particularly acknowledge the contributions from our assistant editors, Catherine Davison, Jessica Bricknell, and George Bundy, who read the entire book and provided us with advice on balance and consistency across the whole endeavour.

Notes on online sources. This book makes extensive use of online resources to provide additional information for the reader. The uniform resource locators (URLs) were checked, but they may become corrupted after publication. It should still be possible to access the resources by inserting the title of the resource into an Internet search engine. Versions of documents that change after publication of this book may also be obtained this way.

Martin Bricknell
Richard Sullivan
2025

NOTE

1. SARS caused a global outbreak in 2002–2004; MERS caused an outbreak in the Arabian Peninsula in 2012, in South Korea in 2015, and in Saudi Arabia in 2018; Ebola caused an outbreak in West Africa in 2013–2016 and in the Democratic Republic of the Congo in 2017–2018; and foot-and-mouth disease has caused outbreaks in cattle in multiple countries.

REFERENCE

1. Sphere Association (2018). *The Sphere Handbook: Humanitarian Charter and Minimum Standards in Humanitarian Response*, 4e. Geneva, Switzerland: Sphere Association www.spherestandards.org/handbook.

PART 1

PERSPECTIVES ON GLOBAL HEALTH AND SECURITY

This first part presents different perspectives on the relationship between health and security. It draws on key concepts from the fields of global health, public health, international relations, security studies, international humanitarian law, healthcare ethics, and military ethics. Whilst not comprehensive on any of these fields, the part provides access to these perspectives for students, practitioners, and researchers from each individual discipline so as to strengthen interdisciplinary understanding.

Chapter 1 defines global health and the relationships between determinants of health, health systems, and health services. Chapter 2 discusses security from the three dimensions of human security, state security, and global security, and their relationships with health. Chapter 3 analyses the health impacts of the worst form of insecurity, war. Chapter 4 examines the new topics in globalisation of climate change and human migration as threats to the health of vulnerable populations. Chapter 5 summarises military technologies, how they are designed to kill and maim, and the biomedical sciences of treatment. Chapter 6 summarises international humanitarian law and ethics as constraints on the worst excesses of war and human barbarism. Chapter 7, the final chapter in this part, discusses the term 'global health security' and how this has placed health within the security agenda. Figure P1.1 shows the location of deaths from armed conflict by country in 2023.

After completing this part, the reader will be able to

- Describe the determinants of health, the components of a health system, and the health services response to insecurity or crisis.
- Describe the meaning of security from the perspective of individual humans, the nation state, and the global international system.

Handbook of Global Health, Security, and War, First Edition. Edited by Martin Bricknell and Richard Sullivan.
© 2025 John Wiley & Sons Ltd. Published 2025 by John Wiley & Sons Ltd.

Included are deaths of combatants and civilians due to fighting in armed conflicts¹ that were ongoing that year.

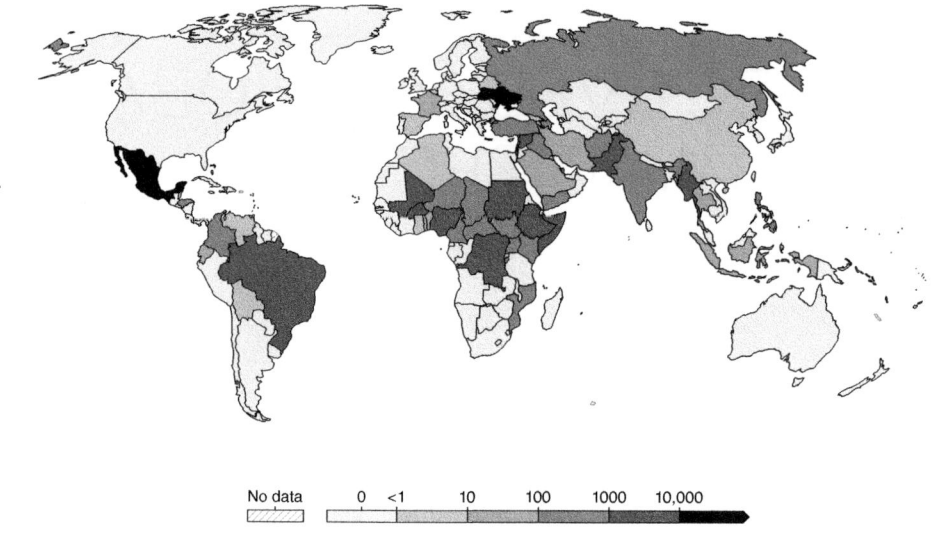

1. Armed conflict (UCDP and PRIO): A disagreement between organized groups, or between one organized group and civilians, that causes at least 25 deaths during a year. This includes combatant and civilian deaths due to fighting, but excludes deaths due to disease and starvation resulting from the conflict.

FIGURE P1.1   Deaths in armed conflicts based on where they occurred, 2023. *Source*: Uppsala Conflict Data Program (2024); Natural Earth (2022) / CC BY 4.0.

- Describe the impact of war on all dimensions of health, health services, and the wider determinants of health.
- Describe the potential impact of new global trends such as climate change and migration on the security and health of affected populations.
- Describe how weapons' technologies are designed to maim and kill and the impact of biomedical innovation to treat the casualties of war.
- Describe how international humanitarian law, military ethics, and healthcare ethics aim to constrain the impact of war on humanity.
- Describe the term 'global health security' and how this has placed health within the security agenda.

CHAPTER 1

An Overview to Global Health and Health Systems

David Ross[1] and Martin Bricknell[2]

[1] Worshipful Society of Apothecaries, London, UK
[2] Centre for Conflict and Health Security, King's College London, London, UK

Abstract

The aim of this chapter is to define global health and the relationships between the determinants of health, health systems, and health services. It will outline the features and variations in the organisation of health systems and provision of health services. The chapter is a summary of health concepts for students and practitioners of international relations and security studies.

Keywords: determinants of health, health systems, health services, emergency response

---

KEY LEARNING OUTCOMES

By studying this chapter, the reader will be able to:

- Define health
- Understand the determinants of health
- Consider the components of a health system
- Understand the range of health services provided by a health system
- Introduce technical concepts and terms in global health

Handbook of Global Health, Security, and War, First Edition. Edited by Martin Bricknell and Richard Sullivan.
© 2025 John Wiley & Sons Ltd. Published 2025 by John Wiley & Sons Ltd.

WHAT IS HEALTH?

The preamble to the Constitution of the World Health Organization (WHO) states[1]:

> *Health is a state of complete **physical, mental and social** well-being and not merely the absence of disease or infirmity. The enjoyment of the highest attainable standard of health is one of the fundamental rights of every human being without distinction of race, religion, political belief, economic, or social condition. The health of all peoples is fundamental to the attainment of peace and security and is dependent on the fullest co-operation of individuals and States. Governments have a responsibility for the health of their peoples which can be fulfilled only by the provision of adequate health and social measures.*

This positivist, human rights approach emphasises the duty of governments to organise national society so that external factors, which influence health (**the determinants of health**), act to support a healthy environment with health services being arranged to meet the health needs of all citizens. To set this statement in context, please complete Learning Activity 1.1.

Learning Activity 1.1   Are You Healthy?

Take a moment to consider if you are healthy. You might have short-term ill health (e.g. an illness such as a chest infection or an injury such as a sprained ankle) or you might be managing a long-term illness (such as asthma, eczema, bowel disease, and mental ill health).

- Does this matter if you are able to undertake the activities that you wish?
- Do you have a physical health condition that requires you to take medication or limit your activities?
- Do you have a mental health condition such as anxiety or depression?
- Does this make you 'unhealthy', or have you learned to manage your condition?
- Do you know anyone with a long-term condition that prevents them from reaching their maximum potential at work or in their personal lives?
- What if you wear glasses or need to take medication on a long-term basis?

Consider if the factors that could improve your health rest with health professionals, your living environment, or are entirely within your control. Now consider the alternative perspective:

- Is it possible to be healthy whilst living with a long-term disability or a life-limiting health condition such as cancer?
- Can someone who has experienced a permanent spinal injury be healthy, even if they have accepted their condition and can self-manage their lives with a support care package?

This elementary philosophical debate is widely used to open educational programs in public and global health. It tests our own assumptions regarding our perception of the meaning 'to be healthy' and introduces the importance of understanding the perspective of those affected by ill health. This is highly relevant when we consider the impact of insecurity or war on the health of affected populations and identify the determinants of health which affect their physical, mental, and social health.

Figure 1.1 summarises an ecological perspective of the term **'determinants of health'**, which covers the internal and external factors that could influence an individual's health. Our genetics determine the basic functions of our bodies. How we develop depends on how our essential needs of food, water, sanitation, and housing are met. Our personal behaviours and lifestyles influence how we live and determine the social context in which we live. If we become ill, we may seek help from health services. All these factors are determined at the macro-level by national government public policy, at a meso-level[2] by community-level influences, and at a local level by personal and family behaviours and resources. This is an easy concept to understand in the abstract but much more difficult to influence in the context of insecurity, conflict, and war. You might consider how these determinants apply in an informal settlement for internally displaced persons fleeing from conflict.

The United Nations (UN) has long been an advocate for development and human rights for all. The UN General Assembly Millennium Summit, held in September 2000, reaffirmed the UN Charter and adopted a series of resolutions that became the Millennium Development Goals (MDGs) to uphold the principles of human dignity, equality, and equity at the global level. In 2016, the MDGs were replaced by the United Nations Sustainable Development Goals (SDGs), that can be considered as a global policy that implements the concept of the 'determinants of health'.[3] These are shown in Figure 1.2. They represent a list of the societal, general socioeconomic, cultural, and environmental factors that influence the three dimensions of health. Each SDG has sub-targets which act to measure progress at a national and global level over time. Unfortunately, SDGs can be substantially damaged for populations affected by insecurity and war. SDG 16, peace, justice, and strong institutions addresses the

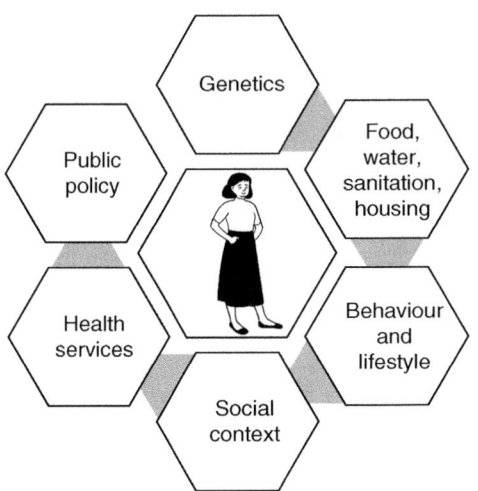

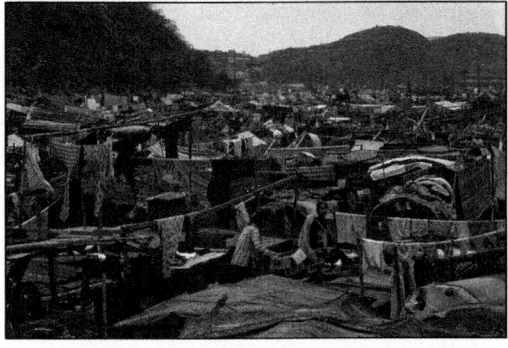

How do these apply in an informal settlement for internally displaced persons?

FIGURE 1.1 Determinants of health.

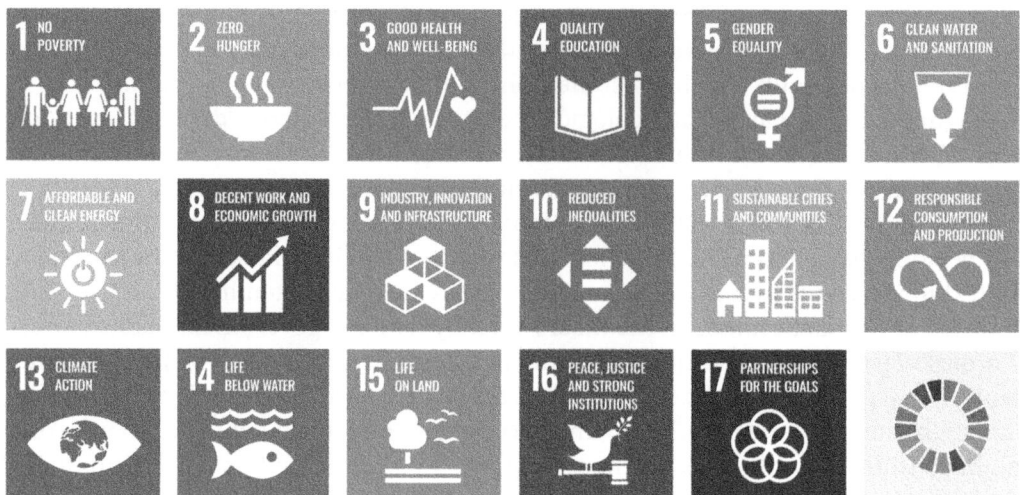

FIGURE 1.2   UN Sustainable Development Goals. *Source*: https://www.un.org/sustainable development/news/communications-material/.

importance of politics and a representational government in setting the leadership for all the other SDGs. The SDGs can also be considered to cover the root causes of threats to **human security**, which will be discussed in Chapter 2.

In 1923, C. E. A. Winslow first defined public health as the science of not only preventing contagious disease but also *'prolonging life, and promoting physical health and efficiency'*. Nowadays, public health is the branch of health science that seeks to address the determinants of health by **p**reventing disease, **p**rotecting health, and **p**romoting healthy lifestyles – the three Ps. Public health practitioners achieve this at the community level through immunisation campaigns, health education, environmental health, and other community and societal efforts. **Global health** applies public health at the global level. Practitioners in global health observe the differences in the determinants of health and health outcomes between countries, at both the regional and global levels. Both public health and global health disciplines emphasise the principles of equity, non-discrimination, and the absence of distinction in access to a healthy environment and the provision of health services as an individual human right. We will return to these principles when we consider the response to a disaster, humanitarian crisis, or complex emergency in Chapter 8.[4]

WHAT IS A HEALTH SYSTEM?

The WHO defines a health system as:

> *'all organizations, people and actions whose primary intent is to promote, restore, or maintain health'* [1]

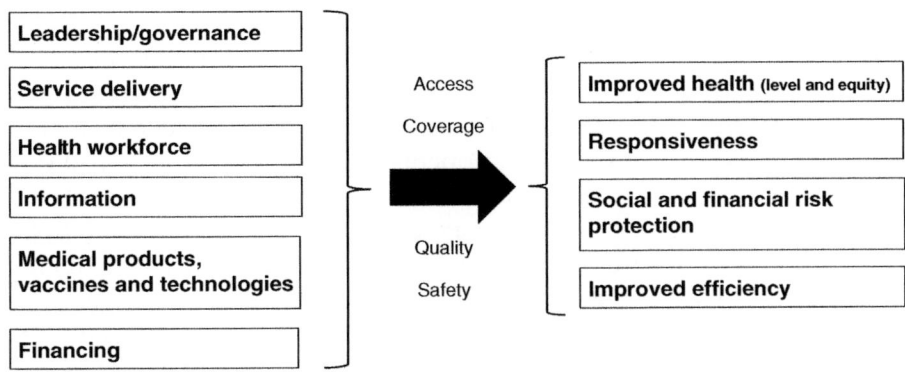

FIGURE 1.3   The building blocks of a health system. *Source*: Adapted from https://www.who.int/healthsystems/strategy/everybodys_business.pdf.

There is wide variation in the design and organisation of health systems around the world each balancing the input costs, the organisation and delivery of services, and the output and outcome measures of health for their populations. All variations represent explicit and implicit political choices between personal risk, individual payment, collective coverage, and government responsibility. Many authors use the WHO 6 building blocks framework to conceptualise the components of a health system and to emphasise that it is much more than just the provider of health services. These are shown in Figure 1.3.

Figure 1.3 shows leadership/governance as the first building block, as it is this that sets the arrangements for all the other functions. A health system needs money, people, logistics, and information to resource health services. The size, efficiency and effectiveness of the management of the 'inputs' will set the access, coverage, quality, and safety of the system. The outputs should be improved health, responsiveness (in terms of time to access healthcare and equity of access), protection against catastrophic consequences (finance, work, social status) of ill health, and efficient use of resources. Multiple organisations such as the WHO, the World Bank, the Organisation for Economic Co-operation and Development, and the Commonwealth Fund publish comparisons of health outcomes and health systems between countries (examples of such analyses are provided at the end of the chapter). **Health systems capacity building** is a term used to describe external support to countries to develop the governance and organisation of their health services. It is often funded through the **overseas development assistance** (ODA) budget from foreign ministries or development agencies. Many countries and international organisations have published 'global health strategies' as policy guidance for their contribution to advancing global health.[5]

Chapter 3 will summarise the impact of war on health and health services.

HEALTH SERVICES

The WHO defines health services as:

"service delivery systems that are responsible for providing health services for patients, persons, families, communities and populations in general, and not only care for patients" [2].

The range and provision of 'health services' are often based on a tiered system of care. **Primary care** covers community services up to the level of a doctor-led clinic. Some health systems have 'sub-primary care' levels, such as health posts that are run by non-doctor community health workers. Primary care may also include mental health services, rehabilitation (e.g. physiotherapy), dental care, optometry (testing of eyesight and fabrication of spectacles), pharmacy, midwifery, and community public health (such as immunisation services). **Secondary care** is considered to be the first level of specialist referral, often based in a hospital, which can also provide in-patient care. This will usually include emergency assessment, maternity, child health, general medicine, general surgery, imaging (such as ultrasound and X-ray), and laboratory support. In some health systems, extended health centres can host forward clinics by hospital specialists and provide diagnostic services such as X-ray, ultrasound, and laboratory testing. **Tertiary care** covers regional hospital services for referrals from secondary care for specialist care for conditions such as heart disease, kidney disease, cancer, and complex long-term conditions. Some systems have a fourth level of clinical services, **quaternary** care, that provides regional or national-level specialist care for complex and rare conditions. This tiered structure is illustrated in Figure 1.4. It is often used as a framework for national health strategies, including explicit definitions of the clinical services and drugs authorised for each tier.

In many countries, the Ministry of Health (or equivalent government ministry at the national level) sets health policies but does not actually organise the provision of health services. This may be delegated to provincial or regional governments and funded by local taxation, or there may be a commercial arrangement funded by government or commercial insurance. Where there is no publicly organised funding, individuals may pay for healthcare as 'out-of-pocket' expenses. The term **'universal health coverage'** (UHC) has been developed to represent a commitment towards a minimum standard of access to health services for all countries funded as a community activity to minimise the risks of catastrophic cost. Figure 1.5 provides a model for

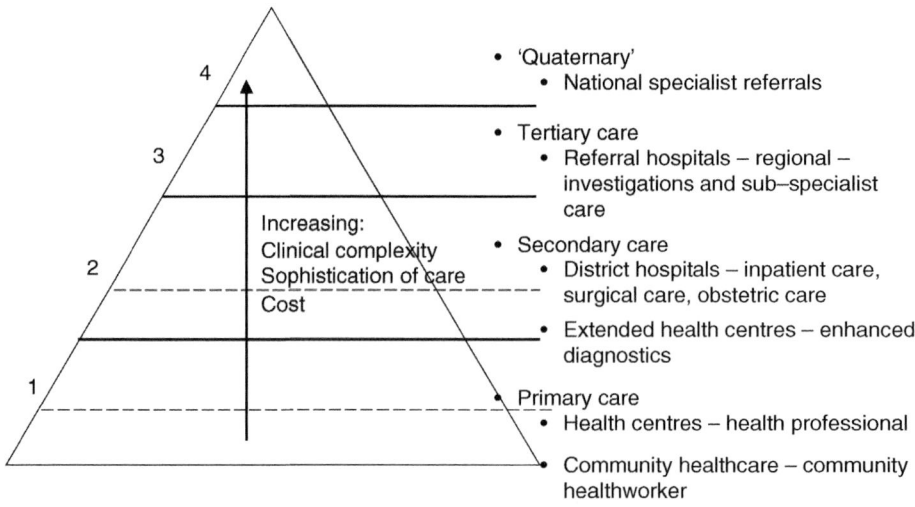

FIGURE 1.4   Levels of healthcare.

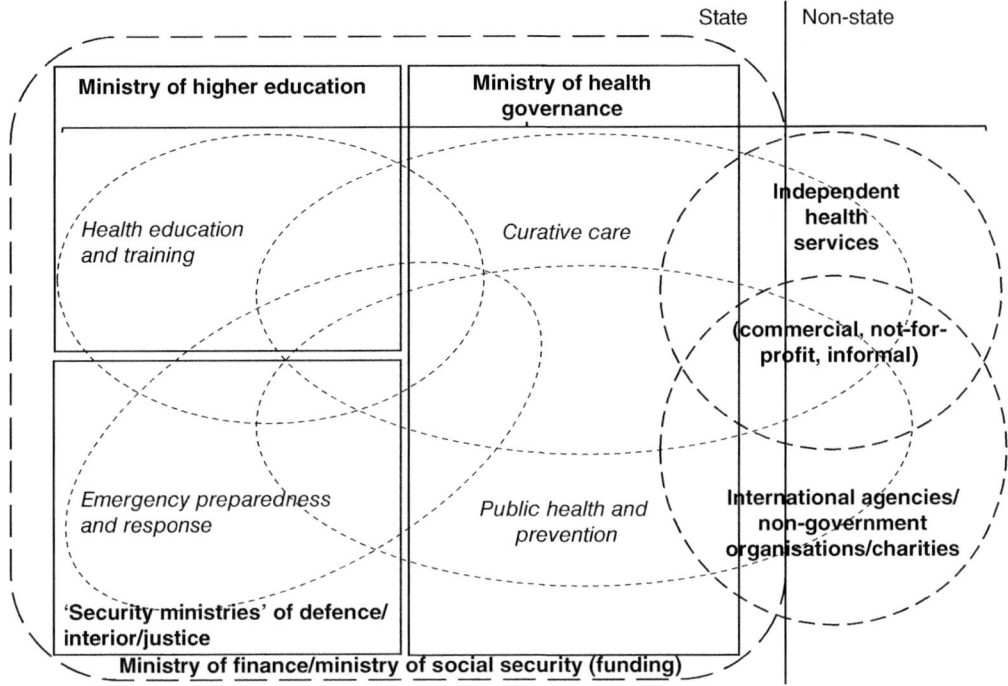

FIGURE 1.5   A country's health service providers.

considering the multiple potential providers of health services in a country, covering government, commercial, and not-for-profit sectors [3].

In principle, state services are funded by the Ministry of Finance through budget allocations to government ministries based on political choices using government income from taxation. In some countries, compulsory contributions to social security funds may be managed separately from taxation income, and so the Ministry of Social Security is also shown as a source of government funding. External donors may also provide direct grant support to government ministries. Non-governmental third-party funders (including non-public insurers/lenders) may also provide finance to government-provided hospitals. The model shows five government ministries that potentially provide health services: Ministry of Health, Ministry of Higher Education, Ministry of Defence, Ministry of Interior, and Ministry of Justice. The Ministry of Higher Education may run teaching hospitals affiliated with universities that educate doctors, nurses, and allied health professionals. The Ministry of Defence and Ministry of Interior may provide health services for armed forces personnel, police personnel, their families, and retirees. The Ministry of Justice may be responsible for healthcare inside prisons. There may be even more government organisations providing health services or healthcare benefits in individual countries. Non-state providers lie outside the formal control of the government, though they should be subject to national laws and regulations. These are independent providers (commercial providers, not-for-profit providers, and the informal sector including pharmacists and traditional healers) and the international agency (IA)/non-governmental organisation (NGO)/charity sector. This could also include commercial organisations which have such a large workforce that they provide health services as part of their overall benefits package. In poorly developed countries or countries in conflict, the NGO sector may be a major provider of health services sometimes associated with religious missions. The Ministry of Health is often the focus for stewardship of the health system including the frameworks for regulation of healthcare workers, pharmaceuticals, and medical devices. The relative size of each sector is stylised in Figure 1.5. The size will vary from country to country and on the unit of measure (e.g. dependent population, proportion of nation's health expenditure, and per capita expenditure). The model also shows four types of health services: curative care, public health and prevention, emergency preparedness and response, and health education and training. These types overlap between providers though the principal focus for policy and regulation is likely to lie with a specific government department.

HEALTH SYSTEMS AND SECURITY

Health systems depend on a secure environment in which to function so that access to health services is equitable, without discrimination, and without risk to providers and recipients.

Globally, very few health systems can meet the needs and expectations of the citizens of their respective countries. This results in explicit or implicit **rationing** of healthcare. Explicit rationing may occur through restricting access to care for certain demographic populations (many countries exclude 'illegal' migrants from the public health system), or by excluding certain conditions or procedures ('cosmetic' plastic surgery is often excluded). Implicit rationing may result in waiting lists or delays in accessing care. If a sudden increase in patients occurs as a result of a health emergency, this rationing becomes more explicit as patients will be **triaged** (sorted) on the basis of clinical need.

Most health systems have procedures to expand emergency health services in the event of a **'major medical incident'** in which extraordinary procedures and practices are implemented to respond to the surge in demand from a natural or man-made emergency. At a local level, this will include stopping all routine activity, mobilising off-duty staff, and expanding the space for emergency patients. At a system level, patients may be diverted to other facilities, existing inpatients may be transferred to other hospitals, and staff may be moved from quieter hospitals to augment the staff in the primary receiving hospital. A longer-duration health crisis such as the COVID-19 pandemic or war requires a sustained adjustment to the management of the health system. This will include national-level resource management of hospital beds (especially specialist beds such as intensive care and burns), strategic management of the healthcare workforce (such as bringing forward graduation for students, or facilitating return to work for retirees), oversight and allocation of medical stockpiles, and underwriting unexpected financial expenditure.

The COVID-19 pandemic highlighted the importance of **resilience** in the critical elements of domestic national infrastructure. Many health systems are vulnerable to overloading, and this vulnerability applies to the health system response to all security threats including pandemics and wars. It covers not only the expansion capacity of the civilian health system but also the capacity of the military health system to treat military casualties, the procurement and logistics of key medical commodities (antibiotics and blood are two examples), and the cyber-protection of the health information architecture. This whole response might be codified through a national framework for emergency planning covering **risk assessment** (identifying threats to health and understanding their likelihood), **prevention** (reducing risk through active countermeasures), **preparation**, **detection** of an actual emergency, **response**, and **recovery**. This will be covered in more detail in Chapter 7. Please undertake Learning Activity 1.2 to understand how the concepts in this chapter are applied in practice.

Learning Activity 1.2 Case Study – Read a National Health Strategy

Using a search engine, find a national health strategy for a low-income or conflict-affected country. Scan the contents against the building blocks of a health system. Compare the description of the organisation of health services with the tiers of primary, secondary, and tertiary care. How might this plan be influenced if the providers of care are not from the Ministry of Health but commercial, charities, or non-governmental organisations? What might be the impact of successful implementation of the strategy as experienced by a pregnant mother in an isolated rural village or a senior doctor working in a teaching hospital in the capital city?

Examples of national health strategies are as follows:

South Korea: `https://www.khepi.or.kr/healthplaneng`
Lebanon: `https://www.moph.gov.lb/en/Pages/0/67043/lebanon-natio nal-health-strategy-vision-2030`
Zambia: `https://www.moh.gov.zm/?p=3138`
Uganda: `https://www.health.go.ug/cause/ministry-of-health-strategic-plan-2020-21-2024-25/`
Somalia: `https://moh.gov.so/so/wp-content/uploads/2022/11/Health-Sector-Strategy-Plan-III.pdf`

LOOKING FORWARD

This chapter has provided an overview to health, health systems, and health services. Health has been defined as a positive state covering physical, mental, and social dimensions. Health systems cover all organisations, people, and actions whose primary intent is to promote, restore, or maintain health. Health services can be considered as three tiers: primary, secondary, tertiary, and quaternary. They may be provided by a range of government departments and NGOs. All health systems need to be prepared to respond to emergencies and may be severely tested and damaged during conflict. Chapter 2 will provide an overview to security and how insecurity is mitigated through security policies and the use of all the instruments of national power (including health capabilities). Chapter 3 then examines the impact of the most extreme form of insecurity, war, on health and health systems.

SOURCES AND RESOURCES

Suggested Internet search terms are as follows: 'health system strengthening capacity building'; 'universal health coverage'; 'health equity'; and 'health policy and systems'. Suggested websites for further information are as follows:

United Nations Department of Economic and Social Affairs. SDGs – https://sdgs.un.org/goals. This website is the primary reference for information on the SDGs.

WHO supporting national health policies, strategies, plans – https://www.who.int/activities/supporting-national-health-policies-strategies-plans. This page and subordinate pages provide WHO reference material to support countries to develop their own national health policies, strategies and plans.

World Bank – Health – https://www.worldbank.org/en/topic/health. This link covers the World Bank programme of work to support countries to achieve UHC to provide quality, affordable, and accessible healthcare.

Organisation for Economic Cooperation and Development (OECD) – Health – https://www.oecd.org/health/. This link covers the OECD programme of work to support countries to provide high-performing health systems through policies that use health resources to achieve high-level health outcomes through accessible, efficient, and high-quality healthcare.

Commonwealth Fund – International Health Care System Profiles – https://www.commonwealthfund.org/international. This link covers the work of the Commonwealth Fund to compare health systems between the United States and other high-income nations.

Health Knowledge – https://www.healthknowledge.org.uk/. This is a free, online learning resource in public health. It comprises a textbook, text courses, video courses, and management training.

You might consider reading – The Four Horsemen and the Hope of New Age by Dr. Emily Mayhew. ISBN-13: 9781529401714. This book takes the reader through recent humanitarian crises and global threats by reviewing perspectives from humanitarians, biomedical scientists, veterinarians, historians, and peace negotiators. The narrative is accessible from any professional background and highlights the multiple dimensions of global health, security, and war.

NOTES

1. The preamble to the Constitution of WHO as adopted by the International Health Conference, New York, 19 June – 22 July 1946; signed on 22 July 1946 by the representatives of 61 states (Official Records of WHO, no. 2, p. 100) and entered into force on 7 April 1948. Available at https://www.who.int/about/governance/constitution.
2. Meso – 'middle'.

3. The 17 Goals. United Nations Department of Economic and Social Affairs. Sustainable Development. Available at https://sdgs.un.org/goals.

4. The UK Faculty of Public Health sponsors a free online package of learning resources in public health. Available at https://www.healthknowledge.org.uk/.

5. Examples are as follows: France (2023) at https://www.diplomatie.gouv.fr/IMG/pdf/a5_strategy_global_health_v2_bd_cle49712b.pdf; Netherlands (2023) at https://www.government.nl/documents/publications/2023/03/29/dutch-global-health-strategy; and the European Union (2022) at https://health.ec.europa.eu/publications/eu-global-health-strategy-better-health-all-changing-world_en.

REFERENCES

1. World Health Organisation (2007). *WHO's Building Blocks Framework – Everybody Business: Strengthening Health Systems to Improve Health Outcomes: WHO's Framework or Action*. Geneva: World Health Organisation. https://www.who.int/healthsystems/strategy/everybodys_business.pdf (accessed 25 March 2025).

2. World Health Organisation. *Health Services*. World Health Organisation. https://www.who.int/topics/health_services/en/ (accessed 25 March 2025).

3. Bricknell, M., Hinrichs-Krapels, S., Ismail, S., and Sullivan, R. (2021). Understanding the structure of a country's health service providers for defence health engagement. *BMJ Military Health* 167: 454–456. https://doi.org/10.1136/bmjmilitary-2020-001502.

CHAPTER 2

Perspectives on Security

Zenobia Homan[1] and Martin Bricknell[2]

[1] Centre for Science and Security Studies, King's College London, London, UK
[2] Centre for Conflict and Health Security, King's College London, London, UK

Abstract

While interpretations of security vary widely between different perspectives and priorities, it can usually be defined as being free from, or resilient to, potential harms such as fear, want, or danger. This chapter discusses security from the three perspectives of human security, national security, and global security, and their relationships with health. It introduces some key concepts in international relations, security studies, and peace studies for health specialists. It balances the content of Chapter 1 on global health so that the reader can fuse knowledge from security studies with the biomedical disciplines.

Keywords: security, conflict, war, international relations, complex emergencies, spectrum of conflict, instruments of power

---

KEY LEARNING OUTCOMES

By studying this chapter the reader will be able to:

- Understand the meaning of security from the perspective of individual humans, the nation state, and the global international system.
- Understand the enduring nature and changing character of war and conflict.
- Critically engage with perspectives on the relationship between conflict and health.

WHAT IS SECURITY?

Security can be considered as a positive state of 'harmony', similar to the concept of health from Chapter 1. From one perspective, the overriding meaning of security might be to avoid physical harm, while from another it means to guard. Some people will associate security closely with the military, while others link it to diplomatic negotiation [1]. In all of these cases, to measure insecurity, the **threats** are assessed against the **risk** of their manifestation by balancing the **likelihood** of occurrence with the **impact** of their outcome. Risks are then mitigated by the application of resources to **prevent, prepare, respond, and recover** from such events. The concept of security can be explored by considering the question of '**whose security**?'.

As stated in the introduction, security can be considered from three perspectives: human security, national security, and global security. The United Nations Universal Declaration of Human Rights underpinned the philosophical approach to the post-Second World War consensus in international relations by asserting that the basis of all security is **human security** at the individual and community levels [2]. **National security** depends on a sovereign state's internal resources as sources of power to influence its relationship with external nation states. **Global security** is achieved by harmonious relationships between nation states in the global system underpinned by treaties and conventions that provide the rules-based system of international order. We will consider each in turn. To set this in context, please complete Learning Activity 2.1.

Learning Activity 2.1 Reviewing Global Trackers of War, Insecurity, Humanitarian Emergencies, and Peace

War, insecurity, and peace are global issues. A number of organisations have established information systems to monitor and track these by time and location. Scan the websites of the following organisations to consider these questions:

- What do they measure?
- Why is this information important?
- Who uses this information?
- How could this information affect your understanding of the relationships between global health, security, conflict, and war?

ACLED Conflict Index: https://acleddata.com/conflict-index/
CrisisWatch: https://www.crisisgroup.org/crisiswatch
Fragile States Index: https://fragilestatesindex.org/
Global Peace Index: https://www.visionofhumanity.org/
Legatum Prosperity Index: https://prosperity.com/
SIPRI Military Expenditure Database: https://www.sipri.org/databases/milex
Uppsala Conflict Data Programme: https://ucdp.uu.se/encyclopedia
World Economic Forum Global Risks Initiative: https://www.weforum.org/global-risks/
World Health Organization Global Health Observatory: https://www.who.int/data/gho
World Press Freedom Index: https://gijn.org/tag/world-press-freedom-index/

HUMAN SECURITY

Human security is defined by the United Nations as follows:

> *'an approach to assist Member States in identifying and addressing widespread and cross-cutting challenges to the survival, livelihood and dignity of their people.... Based on this, a common understanding on the notion of human security includes the following: The right of people to live in freedom and dignity, free from poverty and despair....Human Security recognizes the interlinkages between peace, development and human rights, and equally considers civil, political, economic, social and cultural rights....Governments retain the primary role and responsibility for ensuring the survival, livelihood and dignity of their citizens'.*[1]

Human security is considered to be protection from threats in seven dimensions: economic, food, health, environmental, personal, community, and political. This can be summarised as freedom from hardship and poverty as well as anxiety and indignity. As described in Chapter 1, based on the success of the Millennium Development Goals, the United Nations General Assembly adopted the human security approach to the framing of the Sustainable Development Goals.[2]

The concept of human security broadens the traditional 20th-century Western view of security, which focused mainly on international relations between states. The human security perspective recognises that threats to security can operate within states as manifested by internal civil wars and that risks to security can arise from non-state-based threats such as pandemics, climate change, and human migration. It also reinforces the authority, and responsibility, of governments, through politics, to meet the needs of their citizens. Human security also provides a route to place the **humanitarian principles** into the agenda for security actors by asserting the protection of civilians and those responding to the needs of civilians under **International Humanitarian Law** (IHL). However, this perspective carries the risk of 'securitising' the humanitarian principles of **neutrality** and **operational independence** and turning the 'public good' principles of **humanity** and **impartiality** into political objects. This will be discussed further in Chapter 6. This human security perspective also emphasises the deeper contextual causes of insecurity for populations by highlighting the roles of politics, economics, and social protection alongside the 'security institutions (armed forces, police, intelligence, judiciary, and prisons)' in achieving human development.

A recent conflict which demonstrates the concept of human security is the Bosnian War (1992–1995). Survivors from Srebrenica have highlighted the severe threats that civilians faced within their own communities during this time.[3] Noncombatants, particularly women and girls, are uniquely vulnerable to brutal acts of violence in war zones. The principles of human security emphasise protecting individuals from such harm – not just by physical protection from violence but by safeguarding their dignity, mental health, and the social structures that enable individuals to rebuild after trauma [3]. Conflict can fracture communities, turning neighbours into perpetrators of violence and uprooting families from their homes. It can deprive individuals of basic safety, family unity, and self-determination. Accordingly, human security acknowledges the complex, personal tolls that war inflicts on civilians, underlining protection, support services, and empowerment measures that go beyond state-focused security.

NATIONAL SECURITY

It can be said that the first duty of government is to protect the state. Traditional Western security studies lie within the academic discipline of **International Relations** which looks at the role of security policy, armed forces, and organised violence in the protection of the state from external and internal threats. This perspective is underpinned by the concept of the **sovereign state** as the unitary government authority over a country defined by borders and its citizens. The state acts as an independent rational actor in relations between states. States are recognised by their representation at the United Nations and are bound by the Charter of the United Nations not to interfere with the internal authority of other states except under specific circumstances of an external threat by another state.

The definition of a state delimited by a political boundary is subtly different from the concept of a **'nation'** as a population with a shared historical, cultural, and social identity that may not lie solely within a geo-political boundary. Consequently, a state-centric view of security can overlook the complex realities faced by communities where identity, culture, and historical ties extend beyond political boundaries – highlighting the limitations of a strictly territorial approach to security. Conflicts may arise when state policies do not align with the identities and aspirations of the populations within their borders, leading to insecurity ranging from civil strife to humanitarian crises. An example illustrating the distinction between a state and a nation is the case of the Kurds: one of the largest ethnic groups in the world without a formal state, who inhabit regions across Turkey, Iraq, Iran, and Syria. Their security needs are intertwined with issues of autonomy, recognition, and socio-economic development [4].

Some scholars and policymakers will place defence at the heart of national security, using it as the justification for expenditure on security actors (such as armed forces, police, border security, and intelligence services) to protect against external and internal threats. However, broader perspectives of security also recognise the importance of community well-being and social cohesion as integral to stability. **Democratic peace theory** argues that democracies are less likely to go to war than dictatorships, democracies do not go to war with each other, and democratic states make the internal national government system more peaceful. **Civil–military relations** theory argues that civilian political leadership over the armed forces (security institutions) ensures that the state's monopoly over the use of violence remains vested in the benefits to citizens through politics rather than coercion. Sustainable Development Goal 16 (SDG 16) – peace, justice, and strong institutions – addresses the need to promote peace, stability, human rights, and effective governance through the rule of law (RoL) and reduce violence. **Security sector reform** (SSR) is one of the political and technical processes to achieve SDG 16. SSR is often used as a justification for the role of international armed forces and police in peacekeeping and international development.

In many countries, national security policy and strategy follow a formal cycle that is initiated by political direction from the government. For instance, in the United States, the process begins with the National Security Strategy (NSS) [5], which is updated periodically based on evolving security challenges and guides the subsequent National Defense Strategy (NDS) [6]. Similarly, the United Kingdom conducts an integrated review [7] every five years, led by the Prime Minister, which informs security priorities and resource allocation through a Defence Command Paper. These structured processes ensure national security policies remain aligned with political mandates and strategic assessments [8].

The first phase of analysis may seek to identify global trends and themes that represent risks to the stability of the peaceful international system. Security strategy determines the attribution of responsibility for the mitigation of these risks alongside the allocation of resources. These resources can be considered as **instruments of national power**. Traditionally, this was considered from the perspective of matching external threats from foreign actors using the acronym **DIME** – diplomatic, information (covering strategic communications and cyber), military, and economic. Using this model, security policy was considered to be the purview for the government departments covering foreign policy, overseas development assistance, defence, and the allocation of resources by the finance department. With the broadening of the concept of security, the classification of threats has expanded to include natural disasters, internal disharmony, health risks, migration, climate change, and space and cyber as contested environments. The definition of agencies that may be subject to SSR has expanded to include intelligence agencies, internal security agencies (e.g. police and border security), the legal system and prisons. Some authors have expanded the dimensions of national security to a new acronym **MIDFIELD** (military, information, diplomatic, financial, intelligence, economic, legal, and development). The COVID-19 crisis re-emphasised **resilience** as an important dimension of national security reflecting the capacity of government and society to respond and recover from existential shocks. Thus, many contemporary national security strategies are framed as an integrated responsibility of all functions of government to protect the security of the state and its citizens, described by Scandinavian countries as **total defence**.

GLOBAL SECURITY

The term **global security** applies the definition of security to the international system in recognition that a breakdown of security between states can have implications for the security of all states. This perspective is founded upon the role of the United Nations and its subordinate bodies in sponsoring a rules-based international system that codifies standards of behaviour between states.[4] **Globalisation** has led to greater interaction and integration between peoples, commerce, and governments across the world. This process is based on the economic benefits of the cross-border movement of goods, services, technology, and capital, underpinned by rules and regulations that minimise transaction costs while protecting sovereignty. Examples include free trade agreements, freedom of movement, banking standards, extradition treaties, and international tax regulations. Globalisation extends into the transmission of ideas, meanings, and values around the world to share cultural identities. Examples include political ideology, popular music, culinary styles, media, and arts. This has been dramatically enabled by the Internet, social media, and other forms of borderless digital communication. The security of this global system is underwritten by political globalisation through the establishment of inter-governmental organisations at the regional and global levels such as the United Nations, the World Trade Organization, the European Union (EU), the Organisation for Security and Co-operation in Europe, the Organization of American States, the African Union, the Association of Southeast Asian Nations, and the Commonwealth of Independent States. In addition to these multidomain entities, there are security-focussed international alliances such as 'Five Eyes', the North Atlantic Treaty Organization, and the Collective Security Treaty Organization. Alongside these **international agencies** (IAs), there are **international non-governmental organisations** (iNGOs) which exert cross-border political influence or undertake operational humanitarian activities across the world. Examples of iNGOs include Amnesty International, the Bill and Melinda Gates Foundation, Save the Children, and the International Committee of the Red Cross.

Many threats to human and national security act at the global level. The breakdown of inter-state security almost invariably has regional and global implications. Some threats lie out with the individual control of states and require mitigation by collective action, such as climate change, human migration, food security, crime, disinformation, epidemic infectious disease, and terrorism.

TRENDS, THREATS, AND RISK

Many experts and policymakers in international security view the international strategic landscape as increasingly unpredictable and marked by heightened competition among major powers. This is the result of trends within the global system that have the potential to disrupt the stability of relations between states and national security. These include climate change, human migration, breakdown of the rules-based international order, transnational crime, international terrorism, emerging disruptive technologies such as artificial intelligence (AI) and proliferation of weapons of mass destruction (WMD) [9]. These global strategic trends often set the context for the process that develops national security policy. The UK Global Strategic Trends: Out to 2055 document, published in 2024, has a whole section on health.[5] These trends may develop into specific threats to national or global security. The relative salience of each threat can be prioritised by risk (likelihood and impact of the manifestation of this threat). An example of this type of analysis is the Global Risks Report published by the World Economic Forum that was included within Learning Activity 2.1. These risks to national security may be published as a National Intelligence Assessment[6] or National Risk Register[7] with responsibility for mitigating these risks assigned to different government departments.

INSECURITY AND WAR

Clearly, the term 'insecurity' is the opposite of security. Armed forces have increasingly framed their contribution to society as more than just fighting the nation's wars by explaining the breadth of their roles across the 'spectrum of conflict'. This is shown

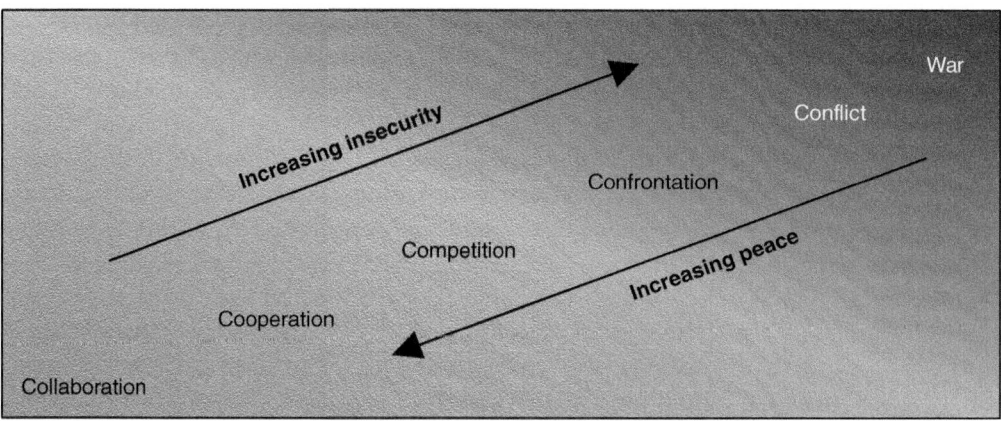

FIGURE 2.1   Spectrum of conflict.

in Figure 2.1. Although peaceful relations between states are the ideal state, it is inevitable that relationships between states (like marriages!) will vary according to political and other factors. Thus, the relationship between states can vary from cooperation to competition, confrontation, conflict, and full-scale war. The starting point depends on whether one perceives war or peace as the primary condition of international relations.

At the most 'peaceful' level, states may actively **collaborate** to achieve mutual benefits. An example might be the **International Health Regulations** [10] in which states agree to share information about infectious diseases and report disease outbreaks to minimise the cross-border impact of outbreaks between states. There are many examples of multi-state **collaboration** in the defence sector such as the co-development and operation of the Eurofighter aircraft by the United Kingdom, Germany, Italy, and Spain. The next level might be **cooperation** in which states work together even if there are limits to the commitment of mutual support. An example might be defensive alliances such as NATO in which all states agree mutual defence commitments in the event of all states being attacked, while the states involved retain national sovereignty over the economics of their defence industries. This is extended into common procedures for the conduct of military operations through Standardisation Agreements (STANAGS). Where the individual interests of states may be different, their behaviour might be more **competitive** in order not to lose comparative advantage. An example might be international trade where a state may wish to protect domestic producers by imposing patents or other protections for intellectual property to prevent their products being copied and sold in the international market. This also applies in the defence industries in which military equipment might be sold between states, but the selling state retains knowledge of key features or restricts key functions. If the relative behaviours of states represent a significant threat to either or both, there might exist a state of **confrontation** in which either or both sides actively contest each other's activities in the international system to ensure no relative disadvantage. An example of confrontation might be the relationship between North Korea and South Korea and their allies in which neither side trusts the other and both sides conduct military exercises to demonstrate their relative potential power. If inter-state relationships deteriorate further, each side may take active measures to harm the other through **conflict** even if either or both sides do not use the full destructive capabilities of their armed forces. An example might be the use of economic and diplomatic sanctions alongside 'deniable' offensive actions in the cyber or intelligence domains as instruments of power in the 'confrontation' between Russia and NATO. Finally, states may undertake active military operations against each other with the purpose of using destructive violence to achieve political aims. This is **war**, though the exact means for the conduct of war might still be constrained in order to limit the extent of mutual destruction. An example might be the 2022 invasion and subsequent war in Ukraine in which neither side has used chemical or nuclear weapons. One might consider the Second World War to have been the only unlimited war in which both sides considered the use of weapons that achieved absolute destruction of all sources of their enemies' instruments of power by attacking economies, industrial production, and the 'morale' of whole populations. Some scholars and policy analysts who are critical of the security perspective claim that 'securitisation' emphasises the risks of insecurity and the importance of mitigating risks of insecurity rather than the benefits of dialogue and co-operation.

The concept of the spectrum of conflict can also apply to the behaviour of states in their approach to relationships in global health. The biomedical science market for drugs and vaccines during the COVID-19 pandemic provides multiple examples. The race to find a vaccine was both collaboration in the exchange of the molecular structure of the virus and co-operation between selected states in the production of candidate vaccines. However, the actual market and distribution became competitive both in the conduct of scientific trials to establish the efficacy of individual vaccines and in the allocation of vaccines to meet the demand by individual states. International sales or donation of vaccines became a source of diplomatic confrontation, with countries like the US and EU members, competing against Russia and China, both seeking to strengthen their influence and build long-term alliances with recipient nations. This extended into active conflict in industrial intelligence as each sought to find classified information on the progress of the other's vaccination programmes. This also applies in the information domain with examples of states conducting active disinformation campaigns to discredit the efficacy of competitors' vaccines and encourage vaccination hesitancy. Fortunately, the COVID-19 pandemic did not result in crossing the threshold of conflict with the active use of destructive military technology between states, though many countries heightened the readiness of their armed forces in case of this eventuality.

The term conflict has been used in the previous section to separate the offensive use of the instruments of national power to achieve relative advantage from their use to actually damage a state's instruments of national power in war. While war can be considered on this spectrum of conflict to be the ultimate extension of power to achieve political aims, it is inherently different because of the use of violent means to harm and destroy an enemy state's resources. In combat, this results in the loss of materiel, such as ships, tanks, and aeroplanes. The conduct of war may extend to causing harm to non-military targets such as buildings, water and sanitation systems, electricity distribution networks and other civilian infrastructures. The ultimate human consequences of war are death, physical injuries, and psychological trauma, which directly affect individuals and societies. This is the enduring **nature of war** [11]. The means to wage war have changed due to developments in military and wider industrial technologies.

The development of bullets, artillery, rockets, aeroplanes, drones, chemical agents, biological weapons, and nuclear bombs all has increased the destructive power of military weapons. The environments for war have extended from the land, sea, and air into space and cyberspace. All of these have changed the **character of war**.

This section has applied the spectrum of conflict to the understanding of security within international relations theories as a relationship between sovereign states acting under the unified control of a government as a controlling actor. These theories can also be applied to relationships between political actors within a state and the concept of '**internal security**'. In a stable society, the government is the dominant security actor and controls the means of security through the police, judiciary, and prisons including the monopoly on the legal use of physical violence. These agencies protect citizens from individuals who choose not to comply with the rules (laws) of the society for their own benefit, such as criminals. While change can emerge from grassroots movements, economic shifts, or cultural developments, politics is often a primary means of enacting societal change by influencing or transforming government policies and leadership. Terrorists might be considered to be individuals who use the means of violence to challenge the internal authority of the state. If the social power of terrorists becomes sufficiently strong, politics, and violence become aligned and the role of government as the unified monopoly holder of the means for violence is broken. The most extreme outcome is civil war. Civil wars are the most barbaric form of war as the political goal is the destruction of the social and legislative authority of the opposition, often resulting in systematic murder, torture, rape, genocide, and forced migration. The term **complex emergency** has been coined to summarise the complexity of providing humanitarian assistance in the absence of unified political authority and government.[8]

PEACE STUDIES

If war is the ultimate form of insecurity, peace could be considered as the ultimate form of security. **Peace studies** can be thought of as an academic discipline which seeks to understand the prevention and resolution of conflict and war. Taking a positivist view, peace, not war, is the natural social condition from the human, national, and global perspectives. Peace is the result of resolution of structural and contextual conditions that motivate the use of violence for political purposes. At the international level, reducing the risks and consequences of conflict and war can be achieved through arms control treaties and other means to attain mutual security through confidence rather than deterrence. The risk of internal conflict can be reduced by removing the tools of violence by disarmament of political groups and controlling the authority for the use of violence through representative civilian government.

The application of these theories can be expressed in the concept of the '**triple nexus**'. In this perspective, humanitarian, development, and peace actors work together to address human security within complex emergencies alongside a political process to create a durable solution to the structural causes of conflict beyond a ceasefire agreement. This places the role of UN multidimensional peacekeeping as provider of human security through implementation of a mandate to establish security; facilitate the political process; protect civilians; assist in the **disarmament, demobilisation and reintegration**

(DDR) of former combatants; support the organisation of elections; protect and promote human rights; and assist in restoring the RoL. External, international peacekeeping forces become the temporary unitary authority for the use of violence by deterring armed actors and restoring security. This provides a safe environment in which emergency humanitarian assistance and longer-term development can meet the needs of populations affected by conflict. This has become codified as **stabilisation operations** in the military doctrine. This explains the use of the military instrument to mitigate crises, promote legitimate political authority, and set the conditions for long-term stability by using comprehensive civilian and military actions to reduce violence, re-establish security, re-establish a **Safe and Secure Environment** (SASE) and RoL, and end social, economic, and political turmoil. This perspective emphasises the trajectory of activities towards the green zone of the spectrum of conflict. The recent World Health Organization (WHO) Global Health and Peace Initiative is an example of the application of peace theories into the practical design of health programmes that can contribute to peace outcomes [12].

HEALTH THREATS AS A RISK TO SECURITY

This book argues that health is an important security topic because threats to health can become risks to security. This is the essence of the emerging discipline of '**global health security**', defined by the WHO as follows:

'the activities required, both proactive and reactive, to minimize the danger and impact of acute public health events that endanger people's health across geographical regions and international boundaries' [13].

Threats to global health include pandemics, antimicrobial resistance (the increasing prevalence of bacteria and fungi to be resistant to all known treatments), the impact of climate change on the global distribution of disease, and misuse of biomedical sciences for warfare (covering biological and chemical weapons). Many commentators have extended the frame of reference to '**One Health**' covering plant, animal, and human health because of the potential for disease to affect food supplies and to cross between species. These topics represent a risk to global security beyond solely public health because the impacts may extend into economic and wider social consequences. Historically, epidemic outbreaks of disease such as plague (Black Death, 14th century in Europe) or influenza (20th-century Spanish influenza) have had global consequences. The WHO was created in 1947 in recognition of the need for international co-ordination in response to disease outbreaks. The WHO 2005 International Health Regulations provides the global treaty that mandates the signatories to report outbreaks of infectious disease. It gives authority to the WHO to declare **public health emergencies of international concern** (PHEIC) if an outbreak of infectious disease constitutes a public health risk to other states through the international spread of disease and to potentially require a coordinated international response. Some countries have developed biosecurity strategies or global health security strategies as components of their wider national security strategies.[9] Global health security will be considered in more detail in Chapter 7 and also as part of the discussion on infectious diseases in Chapter 9.

Many countries include health activities as part of their diplomatic and overseas development strategies. For example, Cuba has long sent medical teams abroad as part of its medical diplomacy, providing healthcare support in Latin America, Africa, and Oceania [14]. '**Global health diplomacy**' is a term used to describe international diplomatic efforts of public health leaders. Chapter 1 introduced the term '**health systems capacity building**' to cover the use of the 'development' instrument of power to improve the effectiveness of external partner countries.[10] Unfortunately, the ultimate consequences of insecurity, conflict, and war are deaths and ill health. We will consider the impact of war on health in Chapter 3. Insecurity also affects access to health services, the capabilities and capacity of health systems, and the clinical health services required to address the health needs of populations affected by insecurity. Part 2 of this book will cover the health services response to crises and these clinical services. Please undertake Learning Activity 2.2 to understand how the concepts in this chapter are applied in practice.

Learning Activity 2.2   Case Study – Read a National Security Strategy

Find an NSS for any country. Scan the contents and consider how the document describes the threats to the country's security, the national sources of power to address these threats, and the allocation of tasks to different government departments to plan and implement the strategy. Then, using a document search tool, find every occurrence for the word 'health' in the strategy and see how it specifically addresses threats to health and mitigates these risks.

Examples of national (international) security strategies:

UK Integrated Review Refresh 2023 at `https://www.gov.uk/government/publications/integrated-review-refresh-2023-responding-to-a-more-contested-and-volatile-world`

US National Security Strategy 2022 at `https://bidenwhitehouse.archives.gov/briefing-room/statements-releases/2022/10/12/fact-sheet-the-biden-harris-administrations-national-security-strategy/`

European Union Strategic Compass at `https://www.eeas.europa.eu/eeas/strategic-compass-security-and-defence-1_en`

Japanese National Security Strategy at `https://www.mofa.go.jp/fp/nsp/page1we_000081.html`

LOOKING FORWARD

This chapter has provided an overview of security theories within the context of global security and applied them to health. It complements the overview of global health theories in Chapter 1. The two together have provided a foundation for our understanding of the relationship between the four words in the book title, 'global', 'health', 'security', and 'war'. Chapter 3 will examine in more detail the health consequences of the most severe form of insecurity, war.

SOURCES AND RESOURCES

Suggested Internet search strings are as follows: 'human security'; 'national security'; 'global trends'; 'global risks'; 'global security'; 'global health security'; 'security sector reform'; 'peace studies'; and 'triple nexus'.

Additional sources are as follows:

United National Trust Fund for Human Security – https://www.un.org/human security/. This website provides a good range of reference resources on the topic of human security.

World Economic Forum Global Risks Initiative – https://www.weforum.org/global-risks/. This website showcases the assessments of the critical global risks facing economies and societies.

Geneva Centre for Security Sector Governance (DCAF) – https://www.dcaf.ch/. The DCAF hosts resources to inform SSR policy and practice in order to make states and people safer through accountable security and justice.

United Nations Peacekeeping Operations – https://www.unmissions.org/. This is the website for all UN missions, including peacekeeping operations, political missions and other political presences. It provides links to UN peacekeeping policies, procedures, and training resources.

NOTES

1. UN General Assembly Resolution A/RES/66/290 10 dated September 2012. Available at https://undocs.org/A/RES/66/290.
2. Transforming our world: the 2030 Agenda for Sustainable Development. United Nations General Assembly Resolution A/RES/70/1 dated 25 September 2015. Available at https://undocs.org/A/RES/70/1.
3. Remembering Srebrenica is a website that memorialises the lessons from Srebrenica to help to build a better, safer and more cohesive society for everyone. Available at https://srebrenica.org.uk/.
4. The UN is an intergovernmental organisation currently composed of 193 member states, each with equal representation in the General Assembly. Key decisions on international peace and security are made by the 15-member Security Council, where five permanent members (the United States, Russia, China, the United Kingdom, and France) hold veto power, and ten rotating members are elected for two-year terms. Votes in the General Assembly carry moral weight, while Security Council resolutions are binding on all UN member states, aiming to uphold a rules-based international order.
5. An example is the UK Global Strategic Trends programme. Available at https://www.gov.uk/government/collections/strategic-trends-programme.
6. An example is the US National Intelligence Community Assessments. Available at https://www.dni.gov/index.php/what-we-do/ic-assessments.

7. An example is the UK National Risk Register. Available at https://www.gov.uk/government/publications/national-risk-register-2023.

8. Definition of Complex Emergencies. Inter-Agency Standing Committee Working Group XVITH meeting on 30 November 1994. Available at https://interagencystandingcommittee.org/sites/default/files/migrated/2014-12/WG16_4.pdf.

9. An example is the second UK Biosecurity Strategy, published in June 2023. Available at https://www.gov.uk/government/publications/uk-biological-security-strategy/uk-biological-security-strategy-html.

10. An example is the UK Global Health Framework published on 22 May 2023. Available at https://www.gov.uk/government/publications/global-health-framework-working-together-towards-a-healthier-world.

REFERENCES

1. Homan, Z., Shaban, Y., and Rane, S. (2022). The language of nuclear security: language diversity in open-source internet searches. *International Journal of Intelligence and CounterIntelligence* 36 (3): 870–891. https://doi.org/10.1080/08850607.2022.2074282.

2. United Nations (1948). Universal Declaration of Human Rights. General Assembly resolution 217 A (III) of 10 December 1948. https://www.un.org/en/about-us/universal-declaration-of-human-rights (accessed 24 March 2025).

3. Gough, M. (2002). Human security: the individual in the security question – the case of Bosnia. *Contemporary Security Policy* 23 (3): 145–191. https://doi.org/10.1080/713999755.

4. Al, S. (2018). Human security versus national security: Kurds, Turkey and Syrian Rojava. In: *Comparative Kurdish Politics in the Middle East* (ed. E. Tugdar and S. Al). Cham: Palgrave Macmillan. https://doi.org/10.1007/978-3-319-53715-3_3.

5. White House (2022). National Security Strategy. https://bidenwhitehouse.archives.gov/briefing-room/statements-releases/2022/10/12/fact-sheet-the-biden-harris-administrations-national-security-strategy/.

6. US Department of Defense (2022). National Defense Strategy. https://media.defense.gov/2022/Oct/27/2003103845/-1/-1/1/2022-NATIONAL-DEFENSE-STRATEGY-NPR-MDR.pdf (accessed 24 March 2025).

7. UK Government (2023). Integrated Review Refresh. https://assets.publishing.service.gov.uk/media/641d72f45155a2000c6ad5d5/11857435_NS_IR_Refresh_2023_Supply_AllPages_Revision_7_WEB_PDF.pdf (accessed 24 March 2025).

8. UK Government (2023). Defence Command Paper. https://www.gov.uk/government/publications/defence-command-paper-2023-defences-response-to-a-more-contested-and-volatile-world (accessed 24 March 2025).

9. For discussion of this label, see Carus, W.S. (2012). Occasional Paper 8, "Defining 'Weapons of Mass Destruction,'" *Center for the Study of Weapons of Mass Destruction*. National Defense University. http://ndupress.ndu.edu/Portals/68/Documents/occasional/cswmd/CSWMD_OccationalPaper-8.pdf (accessed 24 March 2025).

10. World Health Organization (2005). *International Health Regulations.* https://www. who.int/health-topics/international-health-regulations#tab=tab_1 (accessed 24 March 2025).

11. Instability in the context of indiscriminate assault and destruction is timeless. Furthermore, past beliefs, memories and stories form part of the present-day threat landscape. See Homan, Z.S. (2023). Unconventional warfare in the ancient near east. *Social Sciences & Humanities Open* 8: 100501. https://doi.org/10.1016/j.ssaho.2023.100501.

12. World Health Organisation (2019). *WHO Global Health and Peace Initiative (GHPI).* Geneva: World Health Organisation. https://www.who.int/initiatives/who-health-and-peace-initiative (accessed 24 March 2025).

13. World Health Organisation. *Health Security.* Geneva: World Health Organisation. https://www.who.int/health-topics/health-security#tab=tab_1 (accessed 24 March 2025).

14. Feinsilver, J.M. (2010). Fifty years of Cuba's medical diplomacy: from idealism to pragmatism. *Cuban Studies* 41: 85–104. http://www.jstor.org/stable/24487229.

CHAPTER 3

Impact of War on Health

Kiran Attridge[1] and Martin Bricknell[2]

[1] Centre for Health Studies, Worshipful Society of the Apothecaries, London, UK
[2] Centre for Conflict and Health Security, King's College London, UK

Abstract

War has catastrophic effects on individual human, national, and global security. This is most pronounced on human physical, mental, and social health. The aim of this chapter is to provide a framework to consider these effects based on the primary impact of conflict and war on health and health outcomes, the secondary impacts on health systems and services, and the wider tertiary impacts of war on society and their effect on the social determinants of health. It builds upon the general concepts of health that were covered in Chapter 1 and is complemented by Chapter 5 which provides a short review of weapons technologies and how they are designed to kill or maim. The chapters in Part 2 of this book will cover the impact of war on health systems and the demand for clinical services during war in more detail.

Keywords: fragile states, complex emergencies, impact of war, mortality, civilian casualties

---

KEY LEARNING OUTCOMES

By studying this chapter, the reader will be able to:

- Describe the primary impact of conflict on health
- Describe the secondary impact of conflict on health systems
- Describe the tertiary impact of non-health consequences of conflict on the social determinants of health
- Consider how these impacts appear over time and their relationships

---

Handbook of Global Health, Security, and War, First Edition. Edited by Martin Bricknell and Richard Sullivan.
© 2025 John Wiley & Sons Ltd. Published 2025 by John Wiley & Sons Ltd.

POPULATIONS AFFECTED BY CONFLICT AND WAR

The first Learning Activity in Chapter 2 was to review selected online databases and trackers that observe the distribution of insecurity on populations around the world. The term **'fragile and conflict-affected situations (FCASs)'** has been developed by the World Bank to define countries that are either 'fragile'[1] or are in 'conflict'[2] within the list of FCAS-affected countries that is published annually.[3] ReliefWeb is a humanitarian information portal founded in 1996 that is managed by the United Nations Office for the Coordination of Humanitarian Affairs. This hosts a comprehensive suite of data (maps, situation reports, analyses, and other documents) that provides current, critical information on global crises and disasters. The combination of the FCAS list and information from ReliefWeb provides an excellent overview of the populations affected by instability, conflict, and war. Armed actors may be violent criminals, terrorists, warlords, non-state armed groups, or state security forces (police and armed forces). The impact of their violence on populations depends on the physical means that they use to inflict damage on their adversaries. In addition to the use of violence to destroy the opposition's military capability, armed actors may use violence as a coercive measure against populations through the use of tactics which could include systematic killing, rape and sexual violence, forced migration, genocide, and destruction of habitation and food supplies. The detritus of war, **explosive remnants of war (ERW)** (bombs, mines, and booby traps) and chemical contamination of the environment may endure and cause death, injury and ill-health long after the cessation of hostilities.

PRIMARY IMPACTS ON HEALTH

To start this chapter, please undertake Learning Activity 3.1.

This video provides a good insight into the lived, practical realities for populations affected by conflict and war. The civilian population has been denied access to water, food, shelter and the means for a sustainable life. Health facilities have been destroyed, and health professionals have been forced to flee from the region. The civilian population has become internally displaced, living in temporary camps, and vulnerable to outbreaks of preventable infectious diseases. Routine preventive and curative health services have had to be delivered by external agencies such as the United Nations (UN) and international non-governmental organisations (iNGOs) because of the breakdown of local government and the limited effectiveness of national government services.

The primary purpose of weapons is to destroy people and property in order to reduce the material capabilities of the enemy and to undermine their will to resist. Although war is terrible for combatants, civilians have suffered many more deaths from war since 1945 than members of armed groups. Figure 3.1 provides a summary of the military and civilian deaths in modern conflicts and the civilian per cent of the total deaths. In addition to death, conflict and war have a direct impact on the health of populations by causing physical injury, disease and mental trauma. These in turn affect

Learning Activity 3.1   Healthcare in Northern Nigeria

Watch the video available on YouTube: Health Crisis in northeast Nigeria at `https://www.youtube.com/watch?v=WWK7zZzo_dw`

Consider the following questions:

- How many people are affected by the crisis?
- What are the types of crises affecting the population?
- What is the impact on health facilities?
- What are the challenges with accessing healthcare?
- What healthcare interventions are undertaken by the health teams?
- What are the infectious diseases being monitored by the health surveillance system?
- What are the three main killers of under 5 s?

Suggested answers are provided at the end of this chapter.

Major military conflicts						
Conflict	Period	Total deaths	Military deaths	Main foreign army	Civilian deaths	Civilian death rate
Korean war	1950–1953	2,238,172	579,736	33,686	1,658,436	74%
Vietnam war	1965–1974	1,353,000	726,000	58,200	627,000	46%
Persian gulf war	1990–1991	162,341–232,541	20,341–26,541	341	142,000–206,000	87–88%
Balkan war	1991–2001	130,000–140,000	–	–	72,716	52–56%
2nd intifada	2000–2007	5,848	2000	–	3000	51%
Afghanistan	2001–2019	157,052	113,481	2,298	43,571	28%
Pakistan	2001–2019	66,063	41,956	0	24,107	36%
Iraq	2003–2019	276,363–308,212	91,626–100,701	4,572	184,737–207,511	66–67%
Syria/ISIS	2014–2019	179,424	129,572	7	49,852	28%
Yemen	2002–2019	90,072	78,003	1	12,069	13%
Ukrainian	2014–2019	13,117–13,496	9,750–10,129	500	3,367	25–26%

Conflicts with unreliable or missing civilian death numbers are not included, e.g. Yom Kippur, Chechnya, and Iran-Iraq war. (– = Not available).

FIGURE 3.1   The outcome of wars/conflicts in terms of mortality.

the social dimension of health for individuals through their diminished capacity for family life, work, and social engagement with their communities.

Physical injuries from weapons occur as a direct result of damage to biological structures (e.g. skin, bones, blood vessels, and internal organs). Some damage can be repaired, but many war casualties are often left with physical long-term consequences even after the maximum healing has occurred. Disfigurement is common. Amputations, nerve damage, significant tissue defects, and long-term scarring may cause substantial limitations to the residual functioning of the war injured. This is particularly complicated for war-wounded children as their bodies will continue to grow, resulting in the need for frequent adaptation of aids and artificial limbs. Chapter 5 describes how weapons are designed to kill and maim. Chapter 9 describes the clinical services needed to manage the physically injured from war.

War can also cause severe, long-term mental ill health for affected people, whether physically injured or not. The experience of a direct threat to life can cause specific psychiatric conditions such as post-traumatic stress disorder, or it can be the trigger for more common mental ill-health conditions such as anxiety, depression, and substance abuse. The experience of war can also lead to the deterioration of pre-existing mental health disorders, as a result of both direct impact and also the disruption to mental health services and access to medications. The impact of war on mental health services will be considered in more detail in Chapter 13.

SECONDARY IMPACTS ON HEALTH SYSTEMS AND SERVICES

In addition to the primary impact of war on individuals, war can have a catastrophic impact on health systems. Medical facilities may be directly damaged by weapons, resulting in disruption to health service networks, and death and injury to healthcare workers. Cyber-warfare may directly attack medical information systems, leading to the loss of medical records, disruption to the management of clinical services, and the failure of electronic medical devices. There is increasing concern that health personnel, health transports (ambulances), and health facilities are being directly targeted to undermine the morale of military and civilian populations. This may be in direct contravention of **International Humanitarian Law** (IHL) and specific provisions within the **Geneva Conventions** (GCs). The laws of war and the ethical duties of health professionals in conflict and other health emergencies will be discussed in Chapter 6.

War will put pressure on medical procurement and logistic systems by generating unforeseen demands for commodities to treat trauma patients such as stretchers, bandages, intravenous fluids, oxygen, blood, and antibiotics. It is also likely that health protection and public health services will also be affected, resulting in a collapse of disease surveillance, vaccination programmes, and the loss of individual and herd immunity to infectious diseases. This leads to an increased risk of epidemics and loss of capacity to detect and respond to them. War will generate a massive burden of infected open wounds with the potential for antibiotic resistance and contamination of medical facilities with highly resistant bacteria and fungi. This will be considered in Chapters 7 and 10 as part of the discussion on global health security and communicable diseases. Chapter 11 describes the impact of disruption to public health services and immunisation on maternal and child health. This chapter will also consider the health consequences of rape and sexual violence as an instrument of war. The demand for emergency care for injured patients will disrupt other treatment services for long-term conditions such as chronic kidney disease, chronic heart disease, and cancer. The longer-term displacement of clinical activity may result in excess deaths from non-war conditions, similar to that seen in the aftermath of the COVID-19 pandemic. The disruption to the lived environment may result in the adoption of unhealthy lifestyles such as an increase in the prevalence of smoking, eating cheap and malnutritious food, and alcohol or drug abuse, leading to starvation or obesity, and lack of physical exercise. The impact of war on non-communicable diseases will be discussed in Chapter 12.

In addition to the relatively immediate impacts of war on health systems, longer-term effects may exert deeper structural damage. The increased demand for health services is likely to put pressure on the underpinning financial system, leading to delays in paying for services, medical supplies, and salaries. This may result in direct charges to patients and increase the risk of catastrophic out-of-pocket expenses and inflation of costs, undermining any progress towards universal health coverage. It also increases the risk of actual corruption with access to health services becoming a commodity rather than a public good. In addition to death and injury, healthcare workers will also have the challenge of caring for themselves and their families alongside caring for patients. This may prevent them from being available for work if social structures such as childcare and schools are disrupted. Wider economic factors and personal risks may result in migration of healthcare workers, especially those with high-level technical skills who may be able to find work away from the conflict zone. In the short term, it may be possible to mobilise volunteers and fast-track the graduation of health professionals within the health education system. However, the 'brain drain' can create a long-term systemic shortage of healthcare staff because the technical colleges and universities that train the next generation of healthcare workers become devoid of teachers.

TERTIARY IMPACTS ON DETERMINANTS OF HEALTH

The wider effects of war on societies can result in tertiary impacts on the determinants of health. Both direct destruction and the economic damage of war can have consequences on housing, water, power, sanitation systems and food supply. The migration of civilians from the combat zone can put pressure on municipal systems in the receiving communities with formal reception centres and informal camps requiring basic water, sanitation, power, housing, and food services to meet the needs of internally displaced persons or refugees. These settlements may, in themselves, put pressure on measures of societal health (inter-community tolerance, truancy, unemployment, crime) both within the affected groups and also the local host communities. The impact of war on migration will be considered in Chapter 4. War is likely to have wider effects on employment, food production, general education, and measures of social cohesion (such as homelessness, crime, and substance abuse). All of these consequences of conflict act as primary and independent drivers for health inequalities [2]. The weapons of conflict and war can also contaminate the human habitat, preventing the long-term restoration of function for land and the wider environment. ERW such as artillery shells, bombs, booby traps and land mines can make the return to farmland and housing very dangerous and can continue to kill and maim long after the fighting has stopped. This is especially tragic for children who may not be able to identify this risk. The chemical detritus of war can cause genetic damage to subsequent generations with evidence of a link between exposure to nuclear fallout (Second World War atomic bombs dropped on Japan), Agent Orange (US defoliant used during the Vietnam war) and (possibly) depleted uranium (from anti-tank shells used in the Balkans and Iraq), resulting in foetal abnormalities born to mothers exposed to these chemicals.

TIMELINE AND INTERRELATIONSHIPS OF IMPACTS

An indicative timeline for the primary, secondary, and tertiary impacts of war on health is shown in Figure 3.2. The effects of direct harm on individuals and infrastructure are likely to be immediate within the area of actual combat, though artillery, drones, and missiles can extend the range of weapons to make many areas vulnerable to attack. The health system will adjust to the demand for physical trauma services over the short term of a few months by displacing care for many other conditions. This is likely to last for the duration of the actual conflict. The wider impact on retention of health professionals and maintenance of health education programmes may take some time to become manifest, perhaps up to 12 months before having the full effects. If the war endures, then long-term, chronic impacts are likely to become structural after a year or longer as the whole society changes, resulting in the requirement for a comprehensive recovery plan rather than solely a return to the pre-conflict arrangements.

The primary, secondary and tertiary impacts of war on health are interconnected and interact. This can have the effect of compounding the individual impacts and having more serious consequences on quantitative and qualitative measures of health within conflict-affected populations. Research, particularly epidemiological studies, on populations affected by conflict will aggregate measures of ill health at the individual level into rates that record the **incidence** and **prevalence** of measurable health outcomes at the population level. In addition to being a record of individual human suffering, these are also measures of the suffering imposed at the community level by conflict. It is important to use epidemiological tools that record the physical, psychological, and social dimensions of health including those that operate at the socio-political level. These issues will be discussed in Chapter 14 on research in conflict and health. Figure 3.3 is a visualisation of this 'network of causation' based on the ideas of Professor Rita Giacaman [3]. Please undertake Learning Activity 3.2 to understand how the concepts in this chapter are applied in practice.

Time	Immediate	Short-term 0–3 months	Medium-term 3–12 months	Chronic > 1 year
Primary Impact on health	Deaths Injuries Acute mental ill-health	Acute treatment of war injured	Rehabilitation of war injured Development of war related mental health conditions	Recovery of war injured Excess mortality for non-war conditions Outbreaks of vaccine preventable diseases Increase in harmful lifestyles
Secondary Impact on health systems and services	Death and injury to healthcare workers Damage to health facilities Cyber attack Sudden demand for trauma supplies	Disturbance of health procurement and logistics Financial difficulties in health system Displaced clinical services Mobilisation of health volunteers	Migration of healthcare workers Increase in out-of-pocket expenses Antimicrobial resistance	Collapse of healthcare professional education Corruption
Tertiary Impact on determinants of health	Evacuation of population from combat affected areas Damage to civilian infrastructure	Internal displacement Disturbance of government services	Collapse of indigenous food production International migration	Collapse of education system

FIGURE 3.2 Timeline of the impact of war on health.

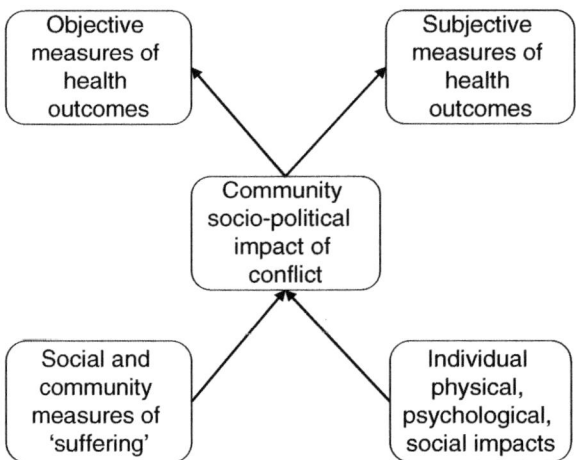

FIGURE 3.3   Network of causation.

Learning Activity 3.2   Case Study – The Syrian Civil War

The civil war in Syria is a multi-sided conflict which started in March 2011 with an attempt to overthrow the regime of President Assad. The protesters gradually formed coherent armed groups, such as the Free Syrian Army, to directly confront the state security forces. In addition to conventional war between the opposing sides, there have been several reports of the use of chemical weapons by the Syrian Armed Forces. By 2015, the regime had lost control of key towns and cities. Russia joined the war in support of the Syrian government in September 2015, and by 2018, most of the territory held by the rebels had been recaptured. Concurrently, the war destabilised Iraq, leading to the formation of the Islamic State group that took key territory in eastern Syria and western Iraq. Kurdish security forces supported by wider Iraqi forces and other international forces defeated the Islamic State and seized territory in northern Syria. Turkey entered the conflict to secure its southern border against Kurdish infiltration. The region was also badly affected by the COVID-19 crisis and a catastrophic earthquake in February 2023. These events have had a devastating impact on health for the Syrian population.

Using Google Scholar (or other academic search engines), search for academic papers using the search string 'syria+war+health+XXXX', where XXXX is one of the following topics: impact, mortality, health system, child, maternal, non-communicable disease, cancer, health systems, health education, pharmaceutical industry, and migration.

Scan the abstract of each paper and note each mention of one of the topics from Figure 3.2. Are any topics covering in the academic literature missing from Figure 3.2?

LOOKING FORWARD

This chapter has provided a summary of the impacts of conflict and war on the health of populations affected by fragile and conflict situations. The classification by primary impacts on health, secondary impacts on health systems and services, and tertiary impacts on determinants of health provides a method for identifying the consequences of war. These can also be expressed over time. Chapter 4 will examine the modern interpretations of the risk of climate change on global security and the specific health needs of internally displaced persons and refugees. Chapter 5 will examine the biomedical effects of weapons of war. Part 2 of the book will look at the health systems' response to health needs arising from conflict.

SOURCES AND RESOURCES

Suggested search strings are as follows: 'war and health'; 'conflict and health'; 'armed conflict and health'; and 'health and peace'.

Additional sources are as follows:

Our World in Data, key insights on war and peace, available at https://ourworldindata.org/war-and-peace. Our World in Data aggregates data from multiple sources to present the best research and data, to make this knowledge accessible and understandable, and to empower those working to build a better world.

ReliefWeb, available at https://reliefweb.int/. This website is a humanitarian information portal hosted by the United Nations Office for the Coordination of Humanitarian Affairs. It is probably the best initial information source on any global crisis or disaster.

Global Humanitarian Overview, available at https://humanitarianaction.info/. The Global Humanitarian Overview is a comprehensive assessment of global humanitarian needs and a forecast of funding requirements across all humanitarian emergencies.

Medact, available at https://www.medact.org/. Medact is an advocacy organisation that conducts research and evidence-based campaigning for solutions to the social, political and economic conditions which damage health, deepen health inequalities and threaten peace and security.

International Physicians for the Prevention of Nuclear War, available at https://www.ippnw.org/. International Physicians for the Prevention of Nuclear War is an international medical organisation dedicated to the abolition of nuclear weapons and the wider prevention of war.

Bulletin of the Atomic Scientists, available at https://thebulletin.org/. The Bulletin of the Atomic Scientists is a non-profit organisation that advocates to raise awareness of the risks to humanity from nuclear weapons, climate change, and disruptive technologies.

Conflict and Health. BMC Journal, available at https://conflictandhealth.biomedcentral.com/. Conflict and Health is an open-access journal that publishes studies which document the public health impacts and responses related to armed conflict, humanitarian crises, and forced migration.

Health and Human Rights Journal, available at https://www.hhrjournal.org/. Health and Human Rights focuses on published academic papers on the conceptual foundations and challenges of human rights and action in relation to health.

Medicine, Conflict and Survival, available at https://www.tandfonline.com/journals/fmcs20. This journal publishes research on the health aspects of violence and human rights and covers topics including consequences of war and group violence and human rights abuse.

Delivering Humanitarian Health Services in Violent Conflicts. Daedalus. Spring 2023. Available at https://www.amacad.org/daedalus/delivering-humanitarian-health-services-violent-conflicts. This is a thematic edition of the journal of the American Academy of Arts and Sciences covering the impact of conflict on vulnerable populations and the dilemmas facing humanitarian health actors.

Learning Activity 3.1   Healthcare in Northern Nigeria – Suggested Answers

- How many people are affected by the crisis?
  Almost 7 million people.
- What are the types of crises affecting the population?
  Food, malnutrition, water – leading to a health crisis.
- What is the impact on health facilities?
  60% of 700 health facilities damaged or destroyed by war.
- What are the challenges with accessing healthcare?
  Distance, security risks.
- What healthcare interventions are undertaken by the health teams?
  Antenatal care, immunisations, treatment for health conditions.
- What are the infectious diseases being monitored by the health surveillance system?
  Cholera, pneumonia, measles …. acute flaccid paralysis (polio), neonatal tetanus, yellow fever, meningitis.
- What are the three main killers of under 5 s?
  Malaria, pneumonia, and diarrhoea.

NOTES

1. 'In a systemic condition or situation characterized by an extremely low level of institutional and governance capacity which significantly impedes the state's ability to function effectively, maintain peace and foster economic and social development'. Classification of Fragility and Conflict Situations. World Bank 2024. Available at https://

thedocs.worldbank.org/en/doc/fb0f93e8e3375803bce211ab1218ef2a-0090082023/original/Classification-of-Fragility-and-Conflict-Situations-FY24.pdf.

2. 'A situation of acute insecurity driven by the use of deadly force by a group – including state forces, organized non-state groups, or other irregular entities – with a political purpose or motivation. Such force can be two-sided – involving engagement between multiple organised, armed sides, at times resulting in collateral civilian harm – or one-sided, in which a group specifically targets civilians'.

3. World Bank. Classification of Fragile and Conflict-Affected Situations. Available at https://www.worldbank.org/en/topic/fragilityconflictviolence/brief/harmonized-list-of-fragile-situations.

REFERENCES

1. Khorram-Manesh, A., Burkle, F.M., Goniewicz, K., and Robinson, Y. (2021). Estimating the number of civilian casualties in modern armed conflicts-a systematic review. *Front Public Health* 28 (9): 765261. https://doi.org/10.3389/fpubh.2021.765261.

2. Bwirire, D., Crutzen, R., Ntabe Namegabe, E. et al. (2022). Health inequalities in post-conflict settings: a systematic review. *PLoS One* 17 (3): e0265038. https://doi.org/10.1371/journal.pone.0265038.

3. Giacaman, R. (2018). Reframing public health in wartime: from the biomedical model to the "wounds inside". *Journal of Palestine Studies* 47 (2): 9–27. https://doi.org/10.1525/jps.2018.47.2.9.

CHAPTER 4

Globalisation, Climate Change, and Migration

Geoff Whitman[1] and Martin Bricknell[2]

[1] Department of Population Health Sciences, King's College London, London, UK
[2] Centre for Conflict and Health Security, King's College London, London, UK

Abstract

The aim of this chapter is to show how globalisation has connected communities across the world by communications, commerce, travel, and knowledge. This has made a significant contribution towards global development, but globalisation also exposes us all to global threats to our security, both natural and man-made. Climate change is perhaps the greatest global threat to the world's habitats for all biological organisms. Rising seawater levels, water scarcity, and extremes of weather may render many current population centres uninhabitable. These factors, plus conflict, have resulted in substantial human migration both within countries and between countries. The chapter will show the impact of these on health.

Keywords: globalisation, climate change, migration, refugee health

---

KEY LEARNING OUTCOMES

By studying this chapter, the reader will be able to:

- Summarise the positive and negative opportunities from globalisation
- Describe the potential impacts of climate change on health
- Describe the impact of internal and external migration on human health

---

DEFINING GLOBALISATION

Chapter 2 provided a brief introduction to the context of global security. It discussed the trends within the international system and identified a series of foundational drivers of change that may create instability and increase the risk of conflict, including: globalisation, climate change, and migration. This chapter will consider how these drivers may also independently affect the determinants of health discussed in Chapter 1.[1] Globalisation can be considered as the process of interaction and integration amongst people, governments, and organisations across the world. This has resulted in the sharing of goods, services, data, technology, culture, political systems, and finance across national borders. It has been facilitated by advances in transportation between countries and over long distances using lorries, trains, ships, and aeroplanes. Advances in communication via the postal system, telegrams, the telephone, faxes, email, mobile phones, and the Internet have widened access to information and knowledge. Both have facilitated the global movement of people, goods and money. Whilst perceived to have been a modern phenomenon of the 19th and 20th centuries, archaeology shows that international trade between empires has been common across millennia. Globalisation can be grouped into three major areas: economic, cultural, and political. Economic globalisation has been facilitated by regional and global trade agreements that set tariffs and taxes, standardise products and services, and formalise the commercial structures that distribute design, production, and logistics according to geographic benefits. Cultural globalisation is the transmission of ideas, values, and knowledge between communities. This has been reinforced by global migration and the impact of social media. Foods, music, and wider arts, sports, religious practice, and many other artefacts of national identity have diffused and penetrated most countries across the world. Political globalisation covers the widening number of international inter-governmental bodies, non-governmental organisations, and advocacy bodies that seek to harmonise international politics and reduce the sovereign, independent power of individual states. In parallel with the opportunities, there is criticism that globalisation is mainly 'Westernisation' from the Global North to the non-Western Global South rather than an equal exchange.

Chapter 2 identified the spectrum of conflict as a concept to explain potential relationships between states from collaboration and co-operation through confrontation and conflict to full-scale war. The two world wars of the 20th century could be considered as the application of globalisation in the conduct of wars across the world's surface. Whilst globalisation is not in its own right a threat to international security, the inter-connectedness and inter-dependencies of most countries can exacerbate the impact of competition, confrontation, conflict, and war across the global system. Please undertake Learning Activity 4.1 to consider the benefits and risks of globalisation.

Learning Activity 4.1 invited you to use the three areas of globalisation as a framework for analysis. An alternative approach might be to consider the impact of globalisation on the concepts introduced in Chapter 1, the determinants of health, and the building blocks of a health system.[2] It could be argued that the greatest

Learning Activity 4.1   Benefits and Risks of Globalisation

Using the three areas of globalisation – economic, cultural, and political – identify some benefits and risks of globalisation for health and health services.
   Some suggested answers are at the end of the chapter.

potential benefit of globalisation for health is at the political level through the agencies of the United Nations (UN). As discussed in Chapters 1 and 2, the Sustainable Development Goals (SDGs) could be considered as a manifestation of the power of the international system to influence states to commit to a human rights approach to meeting the needs of their citizens. The SDGs address many determinants of health and are reinforced by the efforts of global financial institutions, such as the World Bank, to invest in the capacity of countries to meet the SDGs. The World Health Assembly is the international body that represents the health interests of countries. The International Health Regulations 2005 are one example of global cooperation for the protection of global health. Globalisation has created a global market for many of the elements of a health system including global commercial medical companies and health insurance agencies, 'relative freedom of movement' for healthcare professionals, a global supply chain for medical products and devices, exchange of health information and global medical informatics companies, and international collaboration in the conduct of biomedical research, regulation of medical devices, products, professional registration, and internationally accessible health education.

Globalisation can also increase the distribution of threats to the determinants of health. Multinational companies may shift industrial production from highly regulated countries to countries with lower costs and more lenient worker protections. They might actively market harmful products (such as cigarettes, powdered baby milk, and high-calorie refined foods) in developing countries. Supply chains may become vulnerable to political control, shortages, and lack of redundancy. High-income countries may actively recruit health professionals from low-income and low-resourced health systems reducing health capacity in the donor countries. International trade regulations may actively protect high-income countries from market penetration from external suppliers of health products. The primary, secondary, and tertiary impacts of the COVID-19 crisis on health and health services provide an excellent case example of the benefits and risks of globalisation during health crises and will be discussed in Chapter 16.

CLIMATE CHANGE

Climate change is the long-term shift in temperatures and weather patterns. Since the 1800s, human activities have been the main drivers of the sustained increase in global temperatures as a result of the burning of fossil fuels (coal, oil and gas) to generate power [2]. The environmental consequences of climate change are an increasing frequency and severity of extreme storms, sustained droughts, extensive wildfires, rising sea levels, flooding, and disruption of biological habitats. These effects have the potential to affect the lived environment, access to clean water and food, and the risk of natural disasters. As discussed in Chapter 2, most assessments of the risks to global security consider climate change to be a very significant threat due to consequences on the lived environment. This may cause substantial competition for resources (water, food, living space) and consequent tension between communities. Thus, climate change has the potential to have a severe impact on the determinants of health for populations affected by its consequences. Rising temperatures can cause heat illnesses in the very young and elderly amongst communities that cannot afford air-conditioning. Drought and loss of arable land will increase the prevalence of malnutrition. Changes in climate will shift endemic diseases, such as malaria and dengue fever, from the tropics to temperate climates. Extreme weather events such as cyclones and hurricanes will kill people and destroy habitation. All of these events will increase the number of people migrating from vulnerable environments to find safer, more economically sustainable places to live. A comprehensive review of the risks from climate change has been produced by the Lancet Countdown research collaboration [3]. The UK Centre for Climate and Health Security publishes a periodic report on the health effects of climate change in the United Kingdom that is an excellent summary of different effects of climate change on a variety of threats to health [4].

MIGRATION

Globalisation, climate change, and insecurity can be linked as potent underlying causes of human migration. Although migration is an enduring character of human existence, it has become a significant issue of global importance because of the increasing numbers of international migrants causing political and social challenges for both the receiving and departing states. In 2020, it was estimated that there were around 281 million international migrants, approximately 3.6% of the global population [5]. Globally, at the end of 2022, there were 35.3 million refugees, 5.4 million asylum seekers and 71.2 million internally displaced persons with the remainder being economic migrants. This number was greatly reduced during the COVID-19 pandemic. Since 2021, endemic and new conflicts have continued to displace populations in Ukraine, the Occupied Palestinian Territories Syria, Yemen, Afghanistan, the Central African Republic, the Democratic Republic of the Congo, Sudan, Myanmar, and Ukraine. Climate events and natural disasters have displaced populations in China, the Philippines, Bangladesh, India and Haiti.

The UN Migration Agency (International Organization for Migration (IOM)) defines a migrant as follows:

a person who moves away from his or her place of usual residence, whether within a country or across an international border, temporarily or permanently, and for a variety of reasons. The term includes a number of well-defined legal categories of people, such as migrant workers; persons whose particular types of movements are legally defined, such as smuggled migrants; as well as those whose status or means of movement are not specifically defined under international law, such as international students [6].

Proximate causes of migration include seeking work or other opportunities, such as education or human relationships. Populations may be actively 'displaced' as a forced movement due to persecution, conflict, violence, human rights violations and lack of public order. The definition encompasses temporary and permanent movements, within and across borders. Internally displaced persons are people who are forced to leave their home but remain within their country's borders. The 1951 Refugee Convention defines a refugee as a person who:

owing to well-founded fear of being persecuted for reasons of race, religion, nationality, membership of a particular social group or political opinion, is outside the country of their nationality and is unable or, owing to such fear, is unwilling to avail themself of the protection of that country [7].

Migrants may successfully change their place of residence without any adverse consequences. However, migrants may find their journeys very physically and mentally demanding, and they may experience exploitation (including sexual abuse) and persecution. They may have legal and cultural challenges with assimilation in their host community. All of these factors can have substantial consequences for their physical, mental and social health.

THE MIGRATION JOURNEY AND HEALTH

The experience of migration from a usual place of residence may have significant consequences on the physical, mental and social health of the migrant. In addition to the baseline health needs of the individual, their experience across the stages of their journey may influence their health outcomes at their final location. Figure 4.1 summarises the stages and factors that may influence a migrant's health.[3]

Pre-departure: Inevitably, the long-term health of a migrant will be determined by their pre-existing health before departure. This will be influenced by their genetics, age, gender, ethnicity, and socio-economic circumstances. Indeed, seeking access to healthcare might be a motivation for migration in its own right. The actual process of deciding to leave is likely to be stressful, which may have been compounded by persecution, physical violence, torture, or psychological harm.
Transit: The experience of the migrant will be determined by their route, intended receiving country, modes of transport, financial resources, social networks, and the extent of trafficking and exploitation during their journey. This may impose additional exposure to health hazards, stress, and risk. Whilst intermediate countries are obliged by international law to provide support to refugees, this may be limited by political will, resources, or legal jurisdiction.

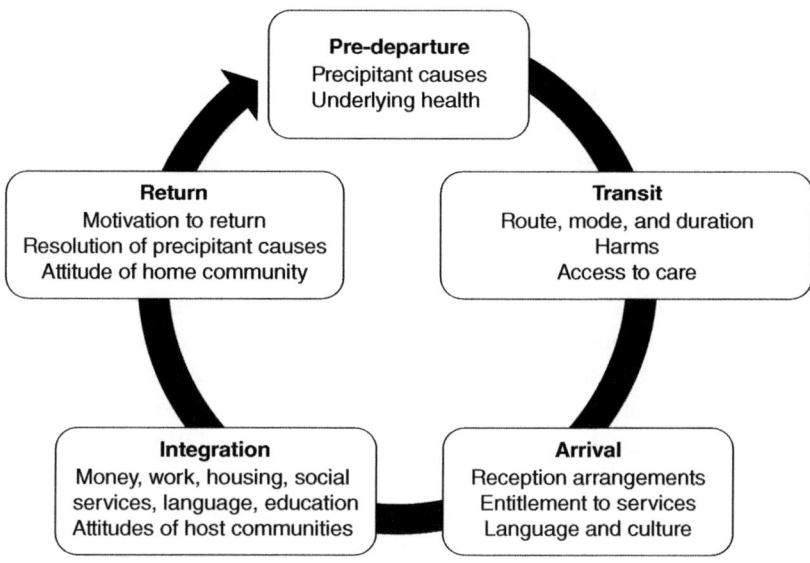

FIGURE 4.1   Factors influencing the health of migrants.

Arrival: The first experience is likely to be the process of registration and information gathering to determine entitlement to stay. This might include an arrival medical examination to detect pre-existing disease and to initiate health protection measures such as vaccinations.

Many countries provide access to health services and social protection for refugees, but this may be incomplete, require out-of-pocket payment, and discriminate by language or behaviours of health professionals. Accessing services may be compounded by cultural differences in the conventions for providing care, understanding of health ideas, and barriers by gender, especially for women. This phase may include holding in a reception or detention centre and restriction of freedom of movement until the authorities have determined the legal status of the migrant. Such reception centres may become a 'de facto' refugee camp if the local authorities prevent the migrants from moving on. International agencies and non-governmental organisations (NGOs) may support the local authorities to establish a formal refugee camp and set up services to meet the essential needs of the migrants, including healthcare. This will be considered further in Chapter 7, Health System Response to Crises.

Integration: In an ideal world, all states would meet the needs of migrants arriving in their country and support them to integrate and establish a new life. However, this is becoming increasingly complex as the number of migrants increases and the topic becomes more politicised in the primary receiving countries. Such policies can have adverse consequences for many of the determinants of health. In some countries, there is a deliberate policy of exclusion and segregation in order to maintain an expectation amongst migrants of returning to their primary country of departure. This may be compounded by restrictions on movement, and limitations to access to health and welfare services, employment, public housing, and education. Migrants can be vulnerable to exploitation, including sexual and gender-based violence. All of these factors can have a detrimental effect on life choices (smoking, alcohol, substance misuse, poor diet, crime), increase the risk of lifestyle-related non-communicable diseases (obesity, diabetes, cardiovascular disease), and permanent damage to their psychological health. These factors may cross into the subsequent generations of migrant families.

Return: An individual's choice regarding permanent migration versus returning home will depend on a wide range of personal, contextual, and political circumstances. Even if a migrant has been granted a long-term right to remain, family and social connections may draw them back to their country of origin. Some countries with large migrant or refugee populations may take active measures to coerce them to return by creating a 'hostile environment' or undertaking active deportation measures. These uncertainties may create additional and enduring psychological pressures.

It is widely accepted that being a migrant carries significant risks to life and health. Many migration routes cross hazardous water or land obstacles that have the potential to kill. The employment conditions for migrant workers may lack the regulatory oversight of mainstream employment, resulting in death and injury from work injuries. Exploitation may extend to violence, especially for women. The living environment may expose them to infectious diseases transmitted by poor water, food, sanitation, crowded accommodation, and sexual behaviour. There may be limitations on accessing healthcare for pre-existing conditions and child and maternal health services. Additionally, the whole migration experience carries significant risks to mental and social health. This is especially important with respect to child mental health and its impact on their education and life chances as an adult. Part 2 of this book will consider the organisation of health services for each of these dimensions of health. Please undertake Learning Activity 4.2 to consider the lived experiences of a displaced family.

Learning Activity 4.2   Case Study – Watch the Video Interview of Migrants at YouTube

Life of a Syrian Family in Islahiye Camp, Turkey – `https://www.youtube.com/watch?v=OENTor011hI`

- What events have the interviewees described that might impact their health?
- What health needs have the interviewees expressed?
- What do you think has happened to them now?

Suggested answers are at the end of the chapter.

LOOKING FORWARD

This chapter has provided an overview to how globalisation and climate change have the potential to affect global health and health systems. We then reviewed migration as a population response to disasters, conflict, and longer-term social and environmental pressures. The provision of services to meet the health needs of migrants is an important dimension of conflict and health because of the dramatic movements of civilian populations during times of insecurity. Their needs should be considered in relation to the stages of their migration journey. Part 2 of this book considers the health services needed during conflict and displacement based on the Sphere Handbook, which is the international reference source for standards in humanitarian response.

SOURCES AND RESOURCES

Suggested Internet search terms are as follows: 'globalisation', 'climate change', 'migration' AND 'security' or 'health' or 'health services'.

Suggested websites and online sources for further information are as follows:

United Nations Climate Action website: https://www.un.org/en/climatechange. This is the primary reference site for information from the United Nations on Climate Change.

The Lancet Countdown on health and climate change. This is an international research collaboration that has produced a series of reports on the impact of climate change on health. The 2023 report is at: Romanello et al. The 2023 report of the Lancet Countdown on health and climate change: the imperative for a health-centred response in a world facing irreversible harms. *The Lancet*. 2023 https://doi.org/10.1016/S0140-6736(23)01859-7.

UN High Commission for Refugees. at https://www.unhcr.org/uk/ and Public Health pages at https://www.unhcr.org/uk/what-we-do/safeguard-human-rights/public-health.

UNHCR Emergency Handbook – Health and Nutrition at https://emergency.unhcr.org/emergency-assistance/health-and-nutrition.

International Organisation for Migration. Migration Health. at https://www.iom.int/migration-health.

Migration data portal at: https://www.migrationdataportal.org/themes/migration-and-health.

World Health Organization. Refugee and Migrant Health Toolkit. at https://www.who.int/tools/refugee-and-migrant-health-toolkit.

Handbook on Refugee Health – https://www.taylorfrancis.com/books/edit/10.1201/9780429464874/handbook-refugee-health-ibrahim-abubakar-alimuddin-zumla-miriam-orcutt-aula-abbara-clare-shortall-sarah-walpole-sylvia-garry-rita-issa and free access at https://www.book2look.com/book/8hqc59wyDv.

Refugee and asylum seeker patient health toolkit. (2019) British Medical Association. Available at https://www.bma.org.uk/advice-and-support/

ethics/refugees-overseas-visitors-and-vulnerable-migrants/
refugee-and-asylum-seeker-patient-health-toolkit.

Globalization and Health – BMC Journal – https://globalizationandhealth.
biomedcentral.com/ This journal publishes research that explores how globalisation processes affect global public health through their impacts on health systems and the social, economic, commercial, and political determinants of health.

Learning Activity 4.1 Benefits and Risks of Globalisation on Health and Health Services – Suggested Answers

	Economic	Cultural	Political
Benefits	Free movement of finance to facilitate global supply chains Free movement of healthcare workers to need shortages Pooling of funds to mitigate crises	Transparency of scientific knowledge and biomedical advances Consensus in approaches to health and health services Multi-centre, multinational research collaborations Medical tourism and travel to access healthcare Increased power and influence of global advocacy organisations	UN and WHO as global fora to advocate for states to address global health issues Transparent information and data sharing for health intelligence Increasing migration and acceptance of refugees
Risks	Vulnerability of complex supply chains to global shocks Exploitation of imbalance of fees and costs between Global North and South Protectionism via tariffs and trade barriers 'Contagion' of consequences of local/regional crises to the whole world Rapid transmission of infectious disease via air travel Increased dominance of multi-national companies with no regulatory controls Marginalisation of disconnected communities	Dominance of Global North biomedical science knowledge and brain drain Cultural expansion of products adverse to global health (cigarettes, processed foods, etc.) Global platforms for socially divisive ideas and movements Multi-national criminal networks	Regression to independence of state sovereignty during global crises Dissemination of disinformation and misinformation Global political institutions controlled by unrepresentative national interests Isolationism and emergence of right-wing groups

Learning Activity 4.2   Case Study – Watch the Video Interview of Migrants at YouTube – Suggested Answers:

- What events have the interviewees described that might impact their health? *This family migrated from Syria due to multiple internal displacements during the war. They witnessed many deaths. The husband is unemployed and expresses frustration at not being able to work. The family has been in the camp for 2.5 years. Many of family were killed in the war, with the remainder living in Lebanon and Beirut. However, some are still in Syria.*

- What health needs have the interviewees expressed? *The husband is blind in right eye and has been taking medicines for 12 years. They clearly expressed social ill health, lamenting the life that they had lost and the challenges of living in limbo in a refugee camp.*

- What do you think has happened to them now? *They are almost certainly still there.*

NOTES

1. You may wish to scan the current edition of the UK Global Strategic Trends programme to see how one analysis identifies these drivers, and others, as a set of dynamics, which will shape the international system for the future, available at https://www.gov.uk/government/collections/strategic-trends-programme.
2. An example of such an integrated analysis is Huynen et al. [1].
3. A very good summary is at Ref. [8].

REFERENCES

1. Huynen, M., Martens, P., and Hilderink, H. (2005). The health impacts of globalisation: a conceptual framework. *Globalization and Health* 1 (1): 14. http://www.globalizationandhealth.com/content/1/1/14.
2. Climate Action. What is Climate Change? United Nations. https://www.un.org/en/climatechange/what-is-climate-change.
3. Romanello, M., Di Napoli, C., Green, C. et al. (2023). The 2023 report of the Lancet Countdown on health and climate change: the imperative for a health-centred response in a world facing irreversible harms. *The Lancet.* 402 (10419): 2346–2394. https://doi.org/10.1016/S0140-6736(23)01859-7.
4. UK Health Security Agency (2024). Health Effects of Climate Change (HECC) in the UK. State of the evidence 2023. GOV-14571. https://www.gov.uk/government/publications/climate-change-health-effects-in-the-uk.
5. McAuliffe, M. and Oucho, L.A. (ed.) (2024). *World Migration Report 2024.* Geneva: International Organization for Migration (IOM) https://worldmigrationreport.iom.int/msite/wmr-2024-interactive/.

6. International Organization for Migration (2019). Glossary on migration, IML Series No. 34, 2019. https://publications.iom.int/system/files/pdf/iml_34_glossary.pdf.

7. UNHCR The 1951 Refugee Convention. https://www.unhcr.org/us/about-unhcr/who-we-are/1951-refugee-convention.

8. World Health Organization (2022). World report on the health of refugees and migrants. Geneva: World Health Organization. https://www.who.int/publications/i/item/9789240054462.

CHAPTER 5

How Weapons Kill

Sohrab Dalal and Martin Bricknell[1]

[1] *Centre for Conflict and Health Security, King's College London, London, UK*

Abstract

The aim of this chapter is to summarise the basic science of weapons, their impact on the human body, and the role of biomedical sciences and industry in both protecting against these threats and developing more efficient means of killing and destruction. The chapter will classify weapons according to the mnemonic **c**hemical, **b**iological, **r**adiological, **n**uclear (CBRN), **e**xplosive, **e**ndemic, **e**nvironmental, and non-battle **t**rauma (CBRNE3T). It will then describe the effects of conventional weapons such as bullets, shells, and bombs on people. The mechanism of action of weapons of mass destruction (WMD) will also be outlined. The chapter will close by considering other emerging weapons technologies and how the effects of some military weapons can be mitigated by protective measures.

Keywords: temporary cavitation, blast injury, CBRN, weapons of mass destruction, left of bang

Sohrab Dalal does not have an affiliation as he wrote this as an independent consultant.

Handbook of Global Health, Security, and War, First Edition. Edited by Martin Bricknell and Richard Sullivan.
© 2025 John Wiley & Sons Ltd. Published 2025 by John Wiley & Sons Ltd.

KEY LEARNING OUTCOMES

By studying this chapter, the reader will be able

- To describe the direct effects of weapons on the human body: explosive, mnemonic chemical, biological, radiological, nuclear (CBRN), environmental, epidemic, non-battle trauma
- To list possible technologies for 'left of the bang' prevention of weapons' injuries

---

INTRODUCTION

Chapter 3 described the primary impacts of conflict on health as death and injuries from weapons. The agents that affect human health during war can be classified using the mnemonic **c**hemical, **b**iological, **r**adiological, **n**uclear (CBRN), **e**xplosive, **e**ndemic, **e**nvironmental, and non-battle **t**rauma (CBRNE3T) [1]. The effects of weapons on the human body depend on the type of weapon and the part of the body that has been attacked. This chapter will consider these agents in turn and describe how they damage the human body. Please complete Learning Activity 5.1 to understand the development of weapons technology in the 20th century.

Learning Activity 5.1   Technological Developments During World War 1

Watch the YouTube Video: Tech Developments of World War I | History – `https://www.youtube.com/watch?v=k7v3cq1ZJjM`
   Consider these questions:

- How were the weapons technologies of World War 1 designed to kill?
- What additional weapons technologies exist in the 21st century to kill?

Suggested answers are at the end of the chapter.

THE EXPLOSIVE AND BALLISTIC EFFECTS OF WEAPONS

So-called conventional weapons cause damage to human tissue by cutting, the transfer of kinetic energy, burns, or explosive energy. Bladed weapons such as knives, swords, and axes cut or tear body tissue causing bleeding, bruising, and damage to structural function (e.g. cutting of nerves and muscles, breaking bones, and damaging internal organs), and allow access to infective organisms to cause abscesses and sepsis. Projectiles such as bullets or shrapnel have the same effects but may cause additional damage through the transfer of energy. Projectiles are classified into low-velocity/low-energy transfer, which causes local tissue damage, and high-velocity/high-energy transfer in which the speed of the bullet transfers kinetic energy to the tissues causing **temporary cavitation** that often results in extensive damage many centimetres distant from the wound track.[1] This temporary cavitation also sucks external contamination deep into the wound risking severe infection unless removed. Military 'anti-personnel' ammunition has developed over the past 200 years to increase velocity and to reduce weight of bullets so that soldiers can carry more, with more destructive power. Ammunition can also be designed to deform (so-called dum-dum bullets), break up, or tumble to increase the transfer of energy from the bullet into the wound.

Explosive weapons (grenades, mortars, mines, shells, bombs, improvised explosive devices) cause additional damage due to the effects of blast. These can be classified into four types as shown in Figure 5.1. **Primary blast injury** is a result of the peak overpressure caused by the actual explosion. This can blow out eardrums, damage the lungs, damage the intestines, shake the brain, and dismember the body. The explosion can also cause thermal burns. **Secondary blast injury** occurs from projectiles displaced by the blast, and these occur either from the weapon itself (e.g. shrapnel or pre-formed fragments from the weapon casing) or from local debris. **Tertiary blast injury** occurs if the blast throws the victim onto other objects. **Quaternary blast injury** covers other mechanisms of injury such as skin burns, inhalation burns, crush injuries, and inhalation of toxic fumes. Nuclear weapons are the most powerful blast weapons. Fuel–air or thermobaric weapons use aerosolised fuel or powdered explosive to maximise the effects of blast. Napalm, phosphorous, and other chemicals can be added to explosive weapons to increase their incendiary effects to use heat to cause damage to humans and physical structures. War surgery is the specific branch of surgery that treats wounds from military weapons and reconstructs the damage to tissues and limbs. This will be covered in Chapter 8 – Physical Trauma. **Non-battle trauma** covers all of the non-weapon

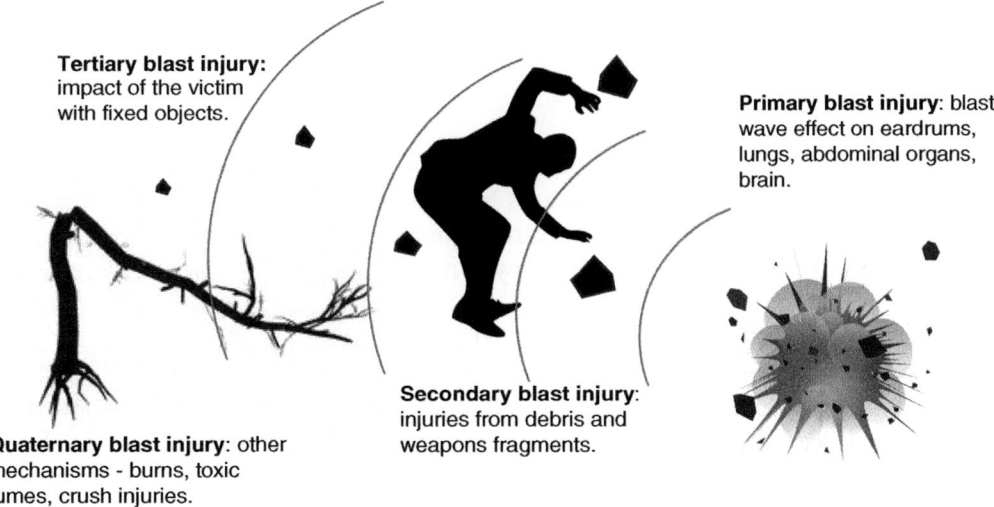

Tertiary blast injury: impact of the victim with fixed objects.

Primary blast injury: blast wave effect on eardrums, lungs, abdominal organs, brain.

Secondary blast injury: injuries from debris and weapons fragments.

Quaternary blast injury: other mechanisms - burns, toxic fumes, crush injuries.

FIGURE 5.1   Types of blast injury.

risks of trauma in a conflict environment such as vehicle, or machinery accidents, falls, or cooking burns.

The damaging effect of bullets and secondary blast injury is directly proportional to the energy transfer from a projectile into the structures of the human body. Within the human body, the amount of energy able to be absorbed without damage is dependent on several factors, including the type and location of tissue. Different tissues can tolerate differing amounts of energy transfer before destructive damage occurs. The energy transfer from a projectile is directly proportional to the mass of the projectile and the square of the velocity of that projectile. The kinetic energy equation is given as follows:

$$K = \tfrac{1}{2}mv^2$$

where K is the kinetic energy, m is the mass of the projectile, and v is the velocity of the projectile.

A doubling of the mass doubles the kinetic energy, but a doubling of the velocity provides four times the kinetic energy and destructive effect. Thus, military bullets and preformed fragmentation weapons (grenades, antipersonnel mines, artillery shells) have become progressively lighter (so more can be carried), while the muzzle velocity of rifles has increased.

Drones and drone swarms can be used to deliver a range of weapons including conventional, chemical, biological, and other munitions. Capitalising on built-in in guidance systems, collective sensing and co-ordinating mechanisms, these have transformed the war in Ukraine. Hypersonic weapon systems are in development across several armed forces. These use hypersonic speeds of over five times the speed of sound to evade missile defences. Unlike conventional trajectory-based ballistic missile systems, hypersonic weapon systems operate at low altitudes and are manoeuvrable in flight onto a target location increasing their effectiveness. These and other emerging weapon delivery systems are likely to bring altered patterns of injury, though they rely on kinetic energy transfer and the four types of blast injury for their effect.

CBRN WEAPONS

CBRN agents are often grouped under the collective term, **weapons of mass destruction (WMD)**. All of these agents have the potential to cause large numbers of casualties and are relatively indiscriminate compared to explosive weapons as their effects can be affected by weather and they can persist in the environment long after their initiation. The military use of WMD and the medical response to CBRN warfare are specialist fields of military medicine. Additional details can be found in the videos at the footnotes or suggested documents in the reading list at the end of this chapter.

Chemical weapons can be standard industrial chemicals (such as chlorine, which causes skin and lung damage), modified industrial chemicals (such as phosgene, which causes severe lung damage), or specially created chemicals (such as persistent nerve agents such as VX and Novichok, which damage nerve control of body functions). Chemical weapons can be categorised by their physiological effect into

blister agents, lung agents, nerve agents, blood agents, and incapacitants (riot control agents and psychological agents). Each type of agent has different symptoms, signs, and potential treatment. The effects of some agents can be reduced by pre-treatment to block the biological action alongside antidotes for post-exposure treatment. Chemical weapons were widely used during the First World War, but were only used by the Imperial Japanese forces during the Second World War. There were multiple uses during the Iraq–Iran war (1980–1988), by Saddam Hussein against the Kurds in 1988, and by government forces during the Syrian civil war between 2012 and 2019. Chemical agents can be dispersed by shells, bombs, sprays, or individual targeting (such as the successful assassination of Kim Jong-nam at Kuala Lumpur Airport in 2017 and the attempted assassination of Sergei and Yulia Skripal in Salisbury, United Kingdom, in 2018).[2]

Biological weapons are naturally occurring organisms (viruses, bacteria, or fungi) or substances derived from organisms, such as toxins, that have been modified as weapons for dispersal and human effects. Biological weapons are relatively cheap to make (compared to the other CBRN agents), but they are difficult to disperse, and their effects are delayed due to the incubation period between exposure and illness, and difficult to constrain once released. The mechanism of effect varies by agent and route of exposure, though this is likely to be very different from naturally occurring disease. It may be possible to reduce the effects of biological agents by taking pre-exposure prophylaxis (e.g. antibiotics or vaccination) or post-exposure treatments (e.g. antitoxins). The development of bioengineering has created a blurring of the separation between chemical and biological warfare, with potential hybrid biochemical compounds being a transitional point between the two types of agents. Genetic modification may also change the infectious characteristics of diseases and make them more effective as biological weapons.[3]

Radiological weapons either use explosive charges to disperse a radioactive source (e.g. as a terrorist device) or are nuclear weapons adapted to maximise the dispersion of radiation rather than blast. Both have the effect of denying access to territory by radiological contamination and by causing fear because of the invisibility and endurance of the hazard. Radiological weapons use the biologically damaging effects of radiation to cause harm by damaging the DNA within cells. Exposure to high doses of radiation causes **acute radiation syndrome (ARS).** The severity of ARS is dependent on the intensity and duration of exposure and affects the ability of cells to function and reproduce. This can cause skin burns, hair loss, failure of blood cell production (red cells, white cells and platelets), failure of intestinal function, and failure of brain function. Medical care for ARS focuses on supporting the failing organs to give them a chance to recover (blood transfusion, antibiotics, and possible stem cell transplant). Lower doses of radiation may cause long-term genetic damage that may result in cancer and birth defects. This is both a dose-related risk and a random risk, and so the long-term impact of radiation exposure for an individual can be difficult to predict.

Nuclear weapons use nuclear fusion or fission to release an immense volume of energy. They cause blast, fire, a radioactive pulse, and radiological contamination of dust, and ash which is dispersed into the atmosphere and then falls back to earth (**nuclear fallout**). Nuclear weapons can be divided into strategic nuclear weapons designed to attack population centres causing such catastrophic damage that the mere threat of use would deter their use in war and limit the political purpose of war. Tactical nuclear weapons have a lower explosive yield and are designed for military use on the battlefield against military targets. However, even this scale of nuclear weapon has the power to damage civilian infrastructure and contaminate a sizeable geographic area of territory. Nuclear weapons have only been used during the Second World War to attack the Japanese cities of Hiroshima and Nagasaki. However, the number of nuclear armed states and weapons has steadily increased since 1945.[4]

ENVIRONMENTAL THREATS

Military personnel and civilians denied access to shelter can be exposed to the environmental extremes of heat and cold. Excessive exposure to high environmental temperatures can cause the body to overheat, resulting in either **heat exhaustion** or **heat stroke**. The risk is increased due to intense physical exercise, wearing of heavy protective equipment, or pre-existing health conditions. Both are medical emergencies that require the patient to be rapidly cooled, rehydrated, and have complications treated. **Cold injuries** result from exposure to cold (and wet) environments. They can be prevented by appropriate protective clothing and shelter. The effects of cold can be divided into localised effects, **frostnip, frostbite**, **non-freezing cold injury (NFCI)**, and systemic effects, **hypothermia**. Both are treated by rewarming of the affected part, and the patient plus general supportive care. **Altitude** is the other military environment which can be a threat to health. Altitude sickness can occur if combat occurs in high mountainous regions, and the effect is compounded by the cold. Altitude, low atmospheric pressure, is a specialist environment for aviation medicine. High atmospheric pressure occurs underwater and is a specialist environment for maritime operations such as diving medicine. Both high and low atmospheric pressures have military dimensions due to the need for armed forces personnel to operate spacecraft, aeroplanes, and submarines. With the identification of space as a new warfare *domain*, the human implications of operating in this environment are a burgeoning area of research and investigation.

EPIDEMIC THREATS

The final category in the CBRNE3T classification of threats to health during war is **epidemic threats**. These are outbreaks of naturally occurring diseases as a result of the breakdown of supplies of safe water and food and the lack of shelter and sanitation, which all increase the risk of transmission of disease. An epidemic occurs when the incidence of a disease in a defined population exceeds that which is normally expected. Historically, many epidemics have been the medium-term consequence of war, such as the Plague of Athens (430 BCE), the Black Death in Europe (bubonic plague, 1347–1351), the Spanish Flu (1918–1919), and cholera in Haiti (2010 onwards). These will be considered in more detail in Chapter 9 – Communicable Disease and Health Security.

EMERGING WEAPON TECHNOLOGIES

This categorisation of health threats during conflict does not include new and emerging military technologies that seek to exploit elements of the electromagnetic spectrum. Lasers have been developed to target the eyes of combatants, which has the potential to be particularly effective against pilots. Microwaves have been investigated as means to cause body discomfort for crowd control. A similar approach has been applied to the security application of sound waves. These 'non-lethal' weapon technologies are particularly attractive for internal security forces to control crowds and civil disturbance without having to resort to more lethal weapons.

Cognitive warfare targets the human mind and its thinking processes, such as memory, thinking, and reasoning. It is associated with emerging and disruptive technologies, such as artificial intelligence, and machine learning as a non-lethal, but weaponised capability focussing on disrupting specific characteristics, such as cognitive biases, of the human condition.

LEFT-OF-BANG PREVENTION

It is possible to mitigate some of the consequences of war by the adoption of protective measures, the so-called **'left of bang'**. This is most obvious in the use of helmets and body armour which have been a long-standing feature of military uniforms. The case for the military helmet was refreshed during the trench warfare of the First World War. Body armour became a standard issue for US forces during the Korean War when a composite nylon waistcoat was shown to substantially reduce injuries from fragmentation weapons. The lower weight of ballistic nylon and ceramics compared to steel plate has made body armour an almost universal issue for armed forces and security forces. Physical protection has been extended to the eyes with ballistic goggles or glasses. Indeed, the whole military uniform can be considered personal protective equipment as it covers the skin (including boots and gloves), is water resistant (or waterproof), and provides insulation against cold. Specialist military uniform is also used to provide protection from skin exposure to chemical weapons. Military-grade gas masks provide protection to the eyes and respiratory system from chemical agents, and inspiration of radioactive dust. The concept of left-of-bang prevention can also be applied to the use of vaccinations to immunise against biological agents (e.g. smallpox and anthrax) or the use of pharmacological pre-treatment in the case of nerve agents or antibiotics as immediate post-exposure prophylaxis against biological agents. Military medical research programmes are investigating other biomedical technologies to protect against traumatic brain injury, prevention of wound infection after injury, and blocking radiation damage to DNA.

Simple 'left-of-bang' human enhancement activities such as diet, hydration, pre-conditioning (both physical and mental), sleep hygiene, and mental well-being are well-recognised 'soft' technologies which provide a protective effect to improve human performance. However, more advanced areas of human enhancement research and capability development include combatant mobility and protection (e.g. using exoskeleton enhancement), cognitive and fatigue mitigation measures, robotics, epi-genetics, bio-electronics and sensors, and human–machine teaming such as brain–computer interfaces. The development of these novel capabilities will push human performance beyond the existing performance envelope, but the resulting effect on human health is poorly understood. Whilst such 'defensive' biomedical sciences research might seem to be ethical, it is important to ensure that the research does not extend into unethical use of biomedical sciences to increase the effectiveness of weapons. The ethical dimensions of weapons development will be considered in Chapter 6. Please undertake Learning Activity 5.2 to understand how international law and conventions have been developed to try to limit the inhumanity of weapons.

Learning Activity 5.2   Case Study – What Treaties and Conventions Exist to Limit the Effects of Weapons?

Using a table based on the CBRNE3T classification, identify international conventions or treaties that seek to limit the effects of weapons on populations.

For example, explosive – 1997 Ottawa Convention or the Anti-Personnel Mine Ban. A completed table is shown at the end of this chapter.

LOOKING FORWARD

This chapter has provided an overview to how weapons kill across the CBRNE3T categorisation of threats to health in war. The chapters in Part 2 cover the clinical health services which mitigate these threats. The next chapter, Chapter 6 – International Humanitarian Law and Ethics, expands on the information which you have collated in Learning Activity 5.2 and considers the application of International Humanitarian Law and ethics in the conduct of war.

SOURCES AND RESOURCES

Suggested Internet search terms are as follows: 'blast injury', 'war surgery', 'CBRN weapons' (look at each separately) and 'explosive remnants of war'.
Suggested websites and online sources for further information are as follows:
    The ICRC has a long history of providing trauma hospitals in humanitarian emergencies. It has also published many textbooks and other guidance for the care of the war wounded. These three books are excellent summaries of the clinical management of casualties from conflict.

- War Surgery – Working with Limited Resources in Armed Conflict, and Other Situations of Violence Volume 1. (2020) ICRC, Geneva. https://shop.icrc.org/war-surgery-working-with-limited-resources-in-armed-conflict-and-other-situations-of-violence-volume-1-pdf-en.html

- War Surgery – Working with Limited Resources in Armed Conflict, and Other SituationsofViolenceVolume2.(2020)ICRC,Geneva.https://shop.icrc.org/war-surgery-working-with-limited-resources-in-armed-conflict-and-other-situations-of-violence-volume-2-print-en.html
- Blast Trauma Care: Course Manual (2020) ICRC. https://www.icrc.org/en/publication/4500-blast-trauma-care-course-manual

Definitive Surgical Trauma Care (DSTC™) Course. https://www.iatsic.org/DSTC/

https://www.taylorfrancis.com/books/mono/10.1201/9781003258124/manual-definitive-surgical-trauma-care-kenneth-boffard-jonathan-white

Emergency War Surgery 5th Edition. (2018) Ed Cubano MA. Borden Institute, Fort Sam Houston, Texas. https://medcoe.army.mil/borden-tb-ews

Allied Joint Chemical, Biological, Radiological and Nuclear (CBRN) Medical Support Doctrine (2022) AMedP 7. NATO. https://www.coemed.org/files/stanags/02_AJMEDP/AJMedP-7_EDB_V1_E_2596.pdf

Medical Management of CBRN Casualties. (2018) AMedP-7.1 NATO. https://www.coemed.org/files/stanags/03_AMEDP/AMedP-7.1_EDA_V1_E_2461.pdf

The last three documents represent military medical views on the organisational and clinical management of military wounds and CBRN casualties. There are subtle differences between the military and civilian perspectives. The civilian view acknowledges delays in care, the limits of available resources, and the need for long-term care of patients within the same geographic health system. The military view is focussed on clearing the battlefield of casualties through an evacuation chain back to their home nation and the best possible standard of care.

Learning Activity 5.1   Technological Developments During World War 1 – Suggested Answers

- How were the weapons technologies of the First World War designed to kill?
  - *Explosive – bullets, shells, bombs – development of machine guns, tanks, aeroplanes, improved methods of targeting, mobilisation of industrial production*
  - *Chemical warfare – first systematic use of chemical agents for warfare*
- What additional weapons technologies exist in the 21st century to kill?
  - Explosive – development of missiles, drones
  - Nuclear weapons
  - Chemical warfare – more refined agents, e.g. nerve agents
  - Biological warfare – development of specific agents for war – e.g. anthrax
  - New technologies – lasers, sound

Learning Activity 5.2   Case Study – What Treaties and Conventions Exist to Limit the Effects of Weapons? Suggested Answers

Chemical	*1993 – Chemical Weapons Convention (CWC), the Convention on the Prohibition of the Development, Production, Stockpiling and Use of Chemical Weapons and on their Destruction*
Biological	*1972 – Biological Weapons Convention (BWC), or Biological and Toxin Weapons Convention (BTWC)*
Radiological	*No treaty, or convention*
Nuclear	*1970 – Non-Proliferation Treaty, or Treaty on the Non-Proliferation of Nuclear Weapons* *2021 – Treaty on the Prohibition of Nuclear Weapons (not signed by any of the nuclear weapon states)* *Various US/Russia nuclear arms reduction treaties*
Explosive	*1899 – Hague Declaration on the use of expanding (Dum-Dum) bullets* *1980 – United Nations (UN) Convention on Certain Conventional Weapons (CCW), Convention on Prohibitions, or Restrictions on the Use of Certain Conventional Weapons Which May Be Deemed to Be Excessively Injurious, or to Have Indiscriminate Effects. Protocol I restricts weapons with non-detectable fragments, Protocol II restricts landmines, and booby traps, Protocol III restricts incendiary weapons, Protocol IV restricts blinding laser weapons, and Protocol V sets out obligations and best practices for the clearance of explosive remnants of war.* *1997 – Ottawa Convention, the Anti-Personnel Mine Ban Treaty, or Convention on the Prohibition of the Use, Stockpiling, Production, and Transfer of Anti-Personnel Mines and on their Destruction.* *2010 – Convention on Cluster Munitions (CCM)*
Environmental	*1977 – Environmental Modification Convention (ENMOD), formally the Convention on the Prohibition of Military, or Any Other Hostile Use of Environmental Modification Techniques*
Epidemic	*Not applicable, separate from biological weapons*
Trauma	*Not applicable*

NOTES

1. Temporary cavitation can be visualised by firing a high-velocity bullet into a block of gelatine. The effect is shown in the video – Bullet Through Ballistic Gel: https://www.youtube.com/watch?v=dFVtNqBNmC0.

2. A short documentary summarising the history of chemical weapons is at A Century of Chemical Weapons – Syria Chemical Attack | The New York Times. https://www.youtube.com/watch?v=J7KbW8zX6Q0.

3. A short US government information film produced in 1952 providing an overview to biological weapons is at What You Should Know About Biological Warfare (1952). https://www.youtube.com/watch?v=Y4ALYK8c5Yg.

4. A short video produced by the ICRC describes the effects of nuclear bomb; if a nuclear bomb dropped on your city, this is the reality you would face | Ban Nuclear Weapons. ICRC 2019. https://youtu.be/kZzHBzIy6Rk.

REFERENCE

1. Bricknell, M. (2014). For debate: the Operational Patient Care Pathway. *Journal of the Royal Army Medical Corps* 160 (1): 64–69. https://doi.org/10.1136/jramc-2013-000228. Epub 2014 Jan 29. PMID: 24478385.

CHAPTER 6

Law and Ethics in Armed Conflict

Tracy Smart[1] and Martin Bricknell[2]

[1] School of Medicine and Psychology, College of Health and Medicine, The Australian National University, Canberra, Australian Capital Territory, Australia

[2] Centre for Conflict and Health Security, King's College London, London, UK

Abstract

The aim of this chapter is to provide a summary of the key features of International Humanitarian Law (IHL) and ethics as they apply to the provision of healthcare in armed conflict. It reviews the law that authorises the use of military force and those that constrain the use of violence during war. It examines ethics as a codified set of behaviours for both military and medical professionals and identifies specific topics that may cause ethical tensions, particularly for military and humanitarian health practitioners. It considers the limitations of IHL, the potential consequences of these ethical tensions, and the evidence that healthcare workers, transports, and facilities may be directly targeted in some conflicts and wars. Finally, it provides an analytical framework for making ethical healthcare decisions.

Keywords: law, medical ethics, medical rules of eligibility, dual loyalty, healthcare in danger, war crimes

Handbook of Global Health, Security, and War, First Edition. Edited by Martin Bricknell and Richard Sullivan.
© 2025 John Wiley & Sons Ltd. Published 2025 by John Wiley & Sons Ltd.

KEY LEARNING OUTCOMES

By studying this chapter, the reader will be able to:

- Describe the linkage between law, ethics, and morality
- Summarise the law in regard to the use of violence in war
- Consider ethical principles as applied to the military and healthcare professions
- Identify some predictable ethical challenges during the conflict
- Describe an approach to analysing an ethical problem in conflict
- Consider the limitations of IHL in constraining the conduct of war

---

WHAT IS LAW IN WAR?

In earlier chapters, we have discussed health and access to healthcare as a human right; the notion that war or organised violence is an extension of politics directed by political leadership; how insecurity and war can have catastrophic consequences for the health of affected populations; and how the weapons of war are designed to destroy the enemy's means of war, with the consequent potential to cause unlimited harm to humanity. This chapter provides a summary of the key features of International Humanitarian Law (IHL) and ethics as they apply to conflict settings. The intent of IHL, also known in military language as the Law of Armed Conflict (LOAC), is to protect the human rights of noncombatants and provide access to healthcare for those affected by conflict through constraining the behaviours of leaders and armed actors in their application of violence.

Healthcare practice is governed through the intersection of law, ethics, and morality. **Law** prescribes a nondiscretionary course of action. **Ethics** is the set of principles that govern a person's activities or behaviours, often codified by professional regulation. **Morality** is a personal code underpinned by an individual's social, cultural, and religious or spiritual context. Note that it is also possible to do something that is technically legal but ethically or morally ambiguous, and vice versa.

The relationships between law, ethics and morality as a 'frame of reference' are summarised in Figure 6.1. This chapter will focus on law and ethics bounded by the dashed line in the figure. However, it is also important to acknowledge that one's personal perspective will be influenced by one's own moral framework. Variations in personal and cultural moral frameworks may provide a reason for why some perpetrators commit atrocities, war crimes, and genocide.

Even though war could be considered an inevitable sociological activity, there have been multiple attempts over history to limit the destructive effects of war and to exempt the defenceless (including the sick and injured, civilians, children, and noncombatant women) from harm. Please undertake Learning Activity 6.1 to consider who might be protected in war by internationally agreed laws and treaties.

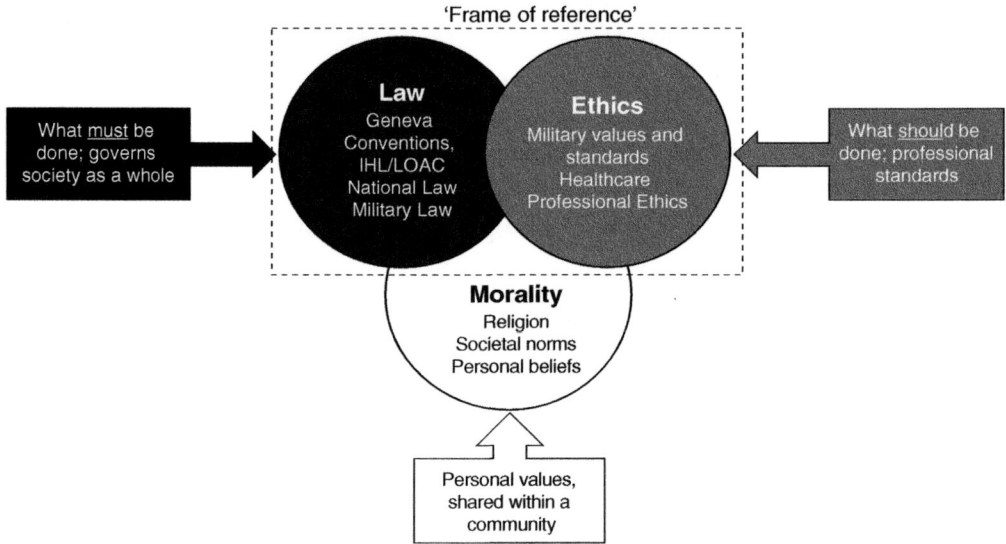

FIGURE 6.1   Law, ethics and morality.

Learning Activity 6.1   What Are the Rules of War?

Watch the YouTube Video: **Rules of War (in a Nutshell) | The Laws of War** (4:44) at `https://www.youtube.com/watch?v=HwpzzAefx9M`

- Who is protected by International Humanitarian Law?
- How are civilians protected under International Humanitarian Law?
- What provisions does International Humanitarian Law make for prisoners or detainees?

The answers are at the end of the chapter.

The legal framework underpinning the use of violence in war is commonly separated into 'jus ad bellum', the legality of states to go to war, and 'jus in bello', the legitimate use of military force during hostilities.

'Jus ad bellum' represents the internal legal processes by which a government is authorised, on behalf of the state, to commit its armed forces to war. This often involves the government obtaining permission from a parliament or other representative body. In international law, Chapter VII of the United Nations Charter recognises the inherent right to self-defence of individual states, or collective groups of states, if an armed attack occurs against a Member of the United Nations, until the Security Council has taken the necessary measures to maintain or restore international peace and security [1]. These laws only apply to 'states'. Non-state armed groups (NSAGs) have no authority in the international system, and there is no legal justification for their use of violence to achieve political outcomes. NSAGs are often classified as terrorists or criminals under national laws.

'**Jus in bello**' covers the laws that apply in war and are guided by LOAC or IHL. The laws are underpinned by four principles: military necessity, distinction, proportionality and humanity. **Military necessity** implies that only legitimate military objectives may be attacked and solely for the purpose of achieving military advantage or defeat of the enemy. **Distinction** ensures that those involved in war, *combatants*, are clearly identifiable from *noncombatants and civilians*. It also requires those controlling weapons to distinguish between them in their attacks. **Proportionality** requires belligerents to make sure that the harm caused to civilians or civilian property (collateral damage) is not excessive compared to the military advantage achieved by the attack. **Humanity** imposes restrictions on the use of weapons that might cause unnecessary suffering or injury relative to their military effect, for example the 1899 Hague Declaration on the use of expanding bullets, cited in Chapter 5. Many countries have a review process to confirm that newly introduced weapons comply with this principle. Military legal advisers view LOAC as seeking to enable the conduct of war within the parameters of the law, whereas the humanitarian community see IHL as constraining the conduct of war by armed actors.

LOAC/IHL is primarily embodied in the Geneva Conventions of 1949 and their Associated Protocols. These commit signatories to avoiding harm to the wounded, shipwrecked, prisoners of war, and civilians. They also make specific provision for the protection and duties of the medical functions of armed forces (personnel, transports, facilities, and units), civil defence organisations, and humanitarian responders. The scope of each convention is summarised in Box 6.1. In addition to the Geneva Conventions, other treaties and international agreements constrain the means for the conduct of war. These were considered in Learning Activity 5.1 in Chapter 5. The 1998 Rome Statute established the International Criminal Court to prosecute individuals accused of war crimes, crimes against humanity, and genocide. This provides legal accountability for individuals who transgress IHL, but it is limited to hearing cases where the offence was committed in a country that is a party to the Rome Statute and where the perpetrator's country of origin had also signed the Rome Statute.

Box 6.1   Summary of the 1949 Geneva Conventions and the 1977 Associated Protocols[1]

Law	Application	Additional explanation
Geneva Convention 1	'For the Amelioration of the Condition of the Wounded and Sick in Armed Forces in the Field'	Covers conduct of war on land
Geneva Convention 2	'For the Amelioration of the Condition of Wounded, Sick and Shipwrecked Members of Armed Forces at Sea'	Covers conduct of war at sea
Geneva Convention 3	'Relative to the Treatment of Prisoners of War'	Covers arrangements for the care and conduct of prisoners of war

(continued)

Box 6.1   (Continued)

Law	Application	Additional explanation
Geneva Convention 4	*'Relative to the Protection of Civilian Persons in Time of War'*	Covers the general protection of civilians and civilian infrastructure, including health facilities
Common 'article 3'	*'Persons taking no active part in the hostilities, including members of armed forces who have laid down their arms and those placed "hors de combat" by sickness, wounds, detention, or any other cause, shall in all circumstances be treated humanely, without any adverse distinction founded on race, colour, religion or faith, sex, birth or wealth, or any other similar criteria'*	
Associated Protocol 1 1977	Additional duties during state-on-state international conflict	
Associated Protocol 2 1977	Additional duties during non-international armed conflict, particularly civil wars	
Associated Protocol 3 2005	Introduces an additional Protective Emblem, the Red Crystal, alongside the Red Cross and the Red Crescent	

MILITARY LAW AND ETHICS

The military profession is unique in that armed forces personnel are authorised to kill on behalf of the state. Military law authorises military commanders to issue such orders and compels subordinates to comply with legal orders. Military law also restricts other rights of citizens when employed within the armed forces such as freedom of speech, the right to withdraw labour, protection of personal information, and other measures necessary for military effectiveness. Military law is also the primary legal format that translates the provisions of IHL into national statutes to give jurisdiction to the national legal system. Many armed forces also proscribe values and codes of conduct that underpin the behaviours of military personnel.[2] These might be considered as equivalent to the ethical frameworks of healthcare practice.

HEALTHCARE LAW AND ETHICS

Across many cultures, there is a long history of prescribing the ethical standards by which doctors and other healthcare professionals practice their art through law or regulation. Medical ethics starts with the dictum **'first do no harm'** ('primum non nocere'). This is reinforced by Beauchamp and Childress's four principles of bioethics:

- **autonomy** (the right of competent adults to determine their treatment),
- **beneficence** and its corollary **non-maleficence** (favourable outcomes for patients with minimal harm) and
- **justice** (treating others equally and fairly) [2].

Many national health professional organisations publish guidance on ethics; however, there is variation in the ethical frameworks of countries' medical bodies. Healthcare ethics has an international dimension, and many global bodies such as the World Medical Association, World Health Organization, United Nations Office for Human Rights, and the International Council of Nurses also publish international guidance.[3]

The challenge of providing healthcare in times of armed conflict while also meeting the needs of the armed forces and other security forces to conduct security operations can cause tensions between military (security) professionals and health professionals. This can be most acute for healthcare workers who serve within the armed forces, a so-called **dual loyalty**. This has been widely debated in the academic literature, with the consensus being that the primary loyalty of healthcare workers is to their profession in keeping with their special status under the Geneva Conventions [3]. Their duties in the armed forces are protected under IHL, and they are prohibited from renouncing these or complying with an illegal order.

SPECIFIC CHALLENGES IN WAR

There has been an increasing concern that the provisions of IHL are being ignored by state signatories[4] and other armed actors with evidence of direct and systematic targeting of healthcare workers, transports, and facilities over the first decades of the 21st century. There have also been suggestions of healthcare workers failing to comply with their duties to protect their patients, specifically in their duties towards prisoners of war. The International Committee of the Red Cross (ICRC) Healthcare in Danger project has attempted to highlight this and reinforce the duties of armed forces personnel and healthcare professionals to comply with IHL [4]. This section considers two specific topics, access to healthcare and the conduct of military health units and military health personnel.

Access to care. The **legal** obligation under IHL requires that armed actors ensure that access to healthcare is solely determined by clinical need. However, individual medical facilities may restrict access on the basis of discrimination by employment, payment coverage, or type of medical condition. During war, there may be differences in the types of patients treated by government hospitals, non-government organisation hospitals, and military hospitals. So-called **Medical Rules of Eligibility** (MRoE)[5] may be applied to describe the groups of patients entitled to be admitted to a military medical facility, particularly on military operations. The 'medical rules of eligibility' are the equivalent of 'eligibility for care' in national health systems, which do discriminate by non-clinical factors such as citizenship, insurance coverage, and employer.

The MRoE for a particular operation will be determined by the mission, the capability and capacity of the deployed health facility, and the capability of the local health system. For instance, forward medical support to a Special Forces mission might have a very light footprint, and so the health personnel will be very constrained as to the type of patients who can be treated. By comparison, a military field hospital deployed to support a response to a humanitarian emergency would normally consider everybody who has been affected by this humanitarian crisis as eligible for admission. The health facility of a humanitarian organisation may explicitly decide not to provide ventilated intensive care beds due to a lack of medical staff or equipment, even though the technology is widely available elsewhere. Additionally, although patients with emergency needs might be entitled to treatment in a specific deployed health facility, the legal requirement in the Geneva Conventions states that parties provide **access to care** according to clinical need. This might mean that the armed forces facilitate civilian organisations to evacuate and care for non-military casualties rather than admit them to military facilities. It is therefore necessary to consider the flow of patients through the whole system (from pre-hospital emergency care all the way through to rehabilitation); the resources available, particularly the bed capacity of the whole system; and finally whether to separate military from civilian healthcare – within the concept of **humanitarian space**. This is an area in which security forces do not operate in order to avoid creating a circumstance where humanitarian actors might be targeted because of perceptions around their involvement with security forces.

The ethical principle that 'health care is to be provided without discrimination' is important in an emergency but does not fully describe the actual ethical duties of healthcare practitioners, particularly in conflict situations, complex emergencies, or humanitarian crises. The ethical obligation of a military healthcare practitioner (MHP) in a clinical setting is to provide emergency care according to clinical need without discrimination if they, and their medical unit, are best placed to do this. It does not place unlimited liability on the whole military health system to care for all patients within a conflict or emergency setting if there are alternative providers, especially for civilians. This means that there may be discrimination between military forces, civilians, and prisoners in who provides the healthcare, but that there is a requirement for all providers of medical care to ensure access and equity across a whole health system.

Conduct of military health units and health personnel. The requirements of military health units and personnel in providing healthcare to victims of armed conflict have been covered. It is this duty, in the spirit of humanitarianism, that confers the rights of protection to both health units and health personnel under the Geneva Conventions. The rights of protection are enshrined in the authority to display the emblems of the Red Cross movement – the Red Cross, the Red Crescent and the Red Crystal. These identify health units and personnel as noncombatants and belonging to the health services, therefore, protected from attack under IHL. Members of the health services of the armed forces have a unique right amongst healthcare workers to carry 'light individual weapons' for the purpose of protection of themselves and their patients. These rights also confer duties and obligations, the most important of which are the obligation not to undertake acts harmful to the enemy, and that military healthcare workers may in no circumstances renounce in part or in entirety the rights secured to them (e.g. by undertaking combatant duties even having removed their Red Cross).

MAKING ETHICAL HEALTHCARE DECISIONS IN WAR

Many ethical challenges during armed conflict and other emergencies do not represent an easy, single, or binary choice. In caring for sick and injured patients in challenging circumstances, military health professionals may experience situations that increase the risk of negative consequences, including mental health issues and '**moral injury**' following exposure. Moral injury has been defined as follows:

> *perpetrating, failing to prevent, bearing witness to or learning about acts that transgress deeply held moral beliefs* [5].

Whether moral injury is distinct from, or a subset of, other conflict-related mental health conditions is not yet evident. Research suggests that pre-deployment preparation, including education and training that allows participants to work through ethically challenging decision-making, and how such decisions could make them feel, may have some protective effect. The same risk factors have also informed the extrapolation of advice to civilian healthcare workers during the recent COVID-19 crisis.

This section describes the use of a Healthcare Ethics Analytical Framework that builds upon the ethical principles previously described and covers perspectives that are framed to include the specific challenges of conflict [6]. It is designed to enable MHPs to reach a decision that complies with the law, their professional standards, and their military duties. It specifically includes the wider perspectives that reflect the nature of healthcare practice in the military environment, including the additional complexity of dual loyalty. The framework can also be used by non-military health professionals. It should be noted that, while training in ethical decision-making using this framework before a deployment or crisis is important, ethical situations may arise on the ground that have not been considered during such training. The framework presented may also be useful when ethical issues arise in real time. For actual use, it is recommended that complex problems are considered by an appropriately experienced team including representatives of the range of clinical professions within a healthcare team, one or more legal advisers, and representatives from the wider community or military command. The process and decision for contentious issues should be formally recorded. The use of this framework is covered in Learning Activity 6.2.

Learning Activity 6.2   Case Study – Analysing Ethical Problems in Health and War

Most frameworks for analysing ethical challenges have the following structure: identification of the issue, analysis including consideration of perspectives, fusion of the analysis, and decision. They tend to focus on clinical decision-making by medical practitioners, rather than explicitly being inclusive of all healthcare practitioners and covering non-clinical ethical dilemmas. The King's Military Healthcare Ethics Analytical Framework follows this generic structure and covers perspectives that are framed to include the societal and military context of war. It is designed to enable military healthcare practitioners (MHPs) and others working in a humanitarian crisis to reach a decision that complies with the law, their professional standards, and their societal/military duties. It comprises four steps:

(*continued*)

Learning Activity 6.2   Continued

STEP 1 – IDENTIFY THE PROBLEM(S)

- Briefly state the scenario
- List the issues that arise from the scenario
- Identify critical information required and assumptions to be made

This step is intended to orientate the decision-making group to the problem and to allow clarification of the problem to determine the exact ethical issues and other consequences. This stage also includes confirmation of critical information required and any assumptions that will form the foundations of the decision.

STEP 2 – ANALYSE

This step considers the problem from four perspectives: patient, clinical, legal and societal/military. This reflects the breadth of perspectives that impact the practice of MHPs within a military context. It is expected that the relative balance of these perspectives will depend on the exact problem. Not every question will be relevant, and additional questions may need to be considered.

1. **Patient**: This quadrant covers the perspectives of patients and their representatives (spouse, wider family, legal advocate). This is the perspective in which Beauchamp and Childress's four principles of ethical healthcare are most likely to apply.
2. **Clinical**: This quadrant covers the perspectives of the clinical team covering all professional groups involved in clinical decision-making. It is also the perspective that should capture any guidance provided by regulatory or professional bodies.
3. **Legal**: This quadrant covers the legal perspective including International Humanitarian Law, national law or military law. In contentious cases, it is recommended that this perspective be provided by a qualified lawyer.
4. **Societal/Military**: This quadrant covers wider, non-clinical perspectives. It includes the ethical perspectives of public health, occupational health, and preventive medicine. This quadrant might also consider if the principle of 'military necessity' gives a 'military commander' the authority to order the military medical services to undertake an activity that would be legal but may not be easy to reconcile ethically (such as a controversial adjustment to Medical Rules of Eligibility).

STEP 3 – FUSE

- Summarise conclusions
- Insert citations to key reference sources for your analysis
- Determine the exact decision(s) to be made

This is the culminating step. The conclusions from the analysis of perspectives should be summarised and key references cited. This will determine the exact decision(s) to be made.

STEP 4 – DECIDE

- What is your decision?
- Why (can you justify it)?
- Residual uncertainly, need for review?

The final step clearly articulates the decision and is the formal record that lists the key reasons for making that decision. This may include a record of areas of enduring uncertainty and any planned review of the decision.

You can now use the framework to analyse a scenario that describes an ethical challenge. You may use the scenarios contained in the Military Healthcare Ethics playing cards that are hosted on the King's Centre for Military Ethics website at `https://militaryethics.uk/en/`

You can also access these via the Military Healthcare Ethics Smartphone App, which you can access for Apple or IOS devices, as per Figure 6.2.

Let us use the MME Card Jack of Hearts to illustrate the use of the King's Military Healthcare Ethics Analytical Framework.

Jack of Hearts – Is it acceptable to allow firearms into a medical facility? If so, who may carry them?

The card is available at `https://militaryethics.uk/en/playing-cards/medical/hearts/j`. Look at the card and review the 'learn more' section or the case analysis provided at the end of this chapter.

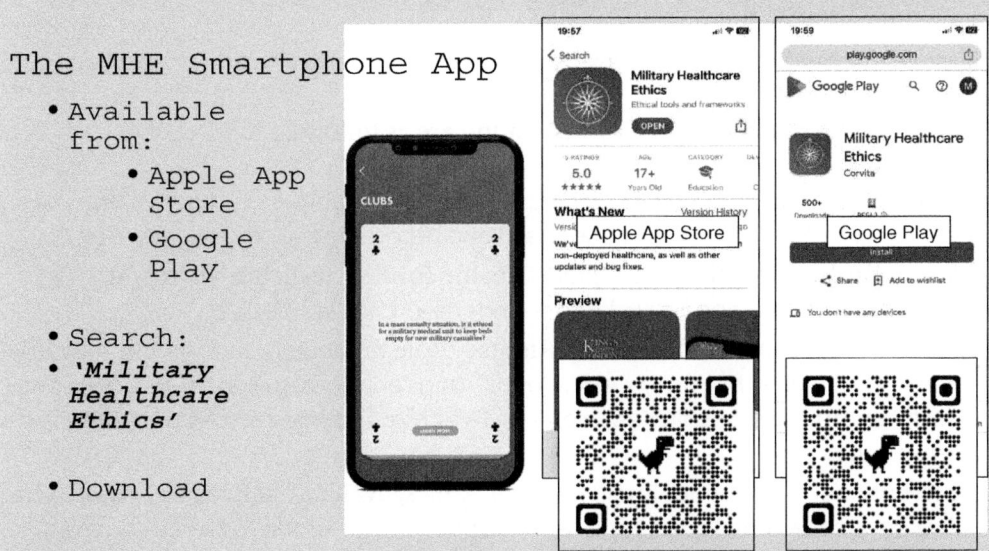

FIGURE 6.2   The Military Healthcare Ethics App.

(continued)

Learning Activity 6.2   *Continued*

Do you agree with the analysis?

Is there anything missing?

Now choose another scenario from the MHE App – Suits: Clubs/Hearts/Spades (Diamonds is about Teamwork). Complete your analysis using the King's Military Healthcare Ethics Analytical Framework from Appendix 1. Please check the 'learn more' section of the card to check that you covered the key points.

LOOKING FORWARD

This chapter provided a short overview of IHL, also known as the law of armed conflict. It considered ethics from the perspective of military and healthcare professionals, recognising that military healthcare professionals may face the challenge of dual loyalty. There are two primary challenges for healthcare during the war: managing access to care and compliance with the rights and responsibilities afforded to healthcare workers, transports, and facilities within IHL. The chapter closed by introducing a framework for analysing ethical challenges in healthcare during conflict and war. The next chapter considers global health security as a specific concept and how mitigation of health threats can be an element of national security policy.

SOURCES AND RESOURCES

Suggested Internet search terms are as follows: 'law and war', 'ethics and war', and 'healthcare ethics and war'.

Suggested websites for further information are as follows:

WMA International Code of Medical Ethics, available at https://www.wma. net/policies-post/wma-international-code-of-medical-ethics/.

World Health Organization Global Health Ethics, available at https://www. who.int/health-topics/ethics-and-health#tab=tab_1.

United Nations Office for Human Rights – Role of Doctors in Protection of Prisoners, available at https://www.ohchr.org/en/instruments-mechanisms/ instruments/principles-medical-ethics-relevant-role-health-personnel.

International Council of Nurses Code of Ethics, available at https://www.icn. ch/resources/publications-and-reports/icn-code-ethics-nurses.

Aid Worker Security Database, available at https://www.aidworkersecurity. org/ – a global compilation of reports on major security incidents involving deliberate acts of violence affecting aid workers.

Relevant books or academic papers are as follows:

ICRC, WMA, ICMM, IFMSA, FIP, and WCPT. Ethical principles of healthcare in times of armed conflict and other emergencies Geneva: ICRC; 2015. Available at `https://www.icrc.org/en/document/common-ethical-principles-health-care-conflict-and-other-emergencies`.

Beauchamp, T.L. *Principles of Biomedical Ethics*. 7th ed. Childress, J.F., editor. New York: Oxford University Press, 2013.

International Committee of the Red Cross (ICRC). The Geneva Conventions and their Commentaries. Geneva. Available at `https://www.icrc.org/en/war-and-law/treaties-customary-law/geneva-conventions`.

ICRC. *Protecting Healthcare: Guidance for the Armed Forces*. Geneva: ICRC; 2020, available at `https://healthcareindanger.org/wp-content/uploads/2021/03/4504_002-ebook.pdf`.

Coupland, R.B., Alex. Health Care in Danger. The responsibilities of health-care personnel working in armed conflicts and other emergencies. Geneva: ICRC; 2020, available at: `https://shop.icrc.org/health-care-in-danger-the-responsibilities-of-health-care-personnel-working-in-armed-conflicts-and-other-emergencies-pdf-en`.

Bricknell, M. and Story, R. An overview to military medical ethics. *Journal of Military and Veterans Health*. 2022;30(2):7–16. Available at `https://jmvh.org/article/an-overview-to-military-medical-ethics/`.

Learning Activity 6.1   What Are the Rules of War? Suggested Answers

Who is protected by International Humanitarian Law?

- *Those not fighting – civilians*
- *Those not able to fight – wounded, sick, prisoners*

How are civilians protected under International Humanitarian Law? Military forces should

- *avoid harming civilians,*
- *not destroy things essential to their survival and*
- *not prevent access to humanitarian support*

(continued)

Learning Activity 6.1   *Continued*

What provisions does International Humanitarian Law make for prisoners or detainees?

- *Prohibits torture*
- *Requires provision of*
  - *Food and water*
  - *Communication to loved ones*

Learning Activity 6.2   Case Study – Analysing Ethical Problems in Health and War

KINGS MILITARY HEALTHCARE ETHICS FRAMEWORK – WORKED EXAMPLE – JACK OF HEARTS

STEP 1 – IDENTIFY THE PROBLEM(S)

- Briefly state the **Scenario – Is it acceptable to allow firearms into a medical facility? If so, who may carry them? MME Cards Jack Hearts**
- List the **Issues** that arise
  - Medical facilities are 'neutral areas' and so firearms should not be present – see ICRC Healthcare in Danger Prevention of entry of weapons into health facilities campaign – https://healthcareindanger.org/no-weapons/.
  - The presence of firearms in a medical facility may cause anxiety to the patients.
  - Firearms may impact the provision of clinical care.
  - 'Anyway – why would anyone wish to care a firearm into a medical facility?'
  - Some patients or visitors may pose a specific threat which has to be mitigated by the presence of armed personnel in a medical facility.
- List **critical information requirements** (CIRs) and **assumptions** to be made
- **CIRs**
  - Why is this question being posed – what is the specific threat, e.g. is the enemy planning to attack a medical facility?
  - Is the facility able to hold weapons in a secure environment? (it may not be practical for very small field medical units to take weapons away from staff/visitors).
- **Assumptions**
  - The question relates to a **military** medical unit, in which medical personnel may be issued with weapons.
  - There is no local threat of direct attack to the unit.
  - The compound in which the medical unit is located is secure.

STEP 2 – ANALYSE

Patient	Legal
What are the views of the patient? (and 'patient group')? How do autonomy, beneficence, non-maleficence and justice apply? Other important factors? Patients should not carry weapons (including outpatients). The patient's environment should be sanitised from military/combat artefacts as much as is reasonable. Personal protective equipment should be available if there is a threat (e.g. helmets, body armour, and gas masks).	Is the scenario covered by IHL including GCs, military law, and other law? Other important factors? Medical units and personnel should be protected and not subject to attack. Geneva Conventions 1, 2, 4 and AP1. ICRC Healthcare in Danger Campaign – prevention of entry of weapons into health facilities – strong humanitarian view that medical facilities should be free of weapons There may be legal rights for designated individuals to carry weapons (e.g. security services and personal security personnel for VIPs)
Clinical	**Societal**
Diagnosis, prognosis, treatment options? Is the scenario covered by professional regulation/guidance? What are the views of the clinical team? Other important factors? Members of the clinical team may have opinions on the carriage of weapons within a medical facility. Personnel with clinical duties should not carry weapons whilst on these duties Clinical staff may refuse to treat patients or to see relatives if they are carrying weapons	Is military necessity involved? Is the scenario covered by military regulation? Is the scenario covered by public health or societal ethics? Other important factors? There may be specific military circumstances where weapons are needed: Part of a medical screening team on a security gate Guarding of prisoners Protection against a definite threat of attack – e.g. 'insider threats' if working within insecure facilities Designated quick response force against attack Carefully consider the implications of military medical personnel visiting civilian medical facilities/meetings, etc., with their personal weapons or senior VIPs visiting the military medical facility

STEP 3 – FUSE

- Summarise conclusions
- Determine the exact decision(s) to be made

(continued)

Learning Activity 6.2   *Continued*

In principle, the clinical areas of a military medical unit should be a 'weapons-free' zone. This requires clear communication. It may be necessary to provide secure storage facilities for weapons if there is a high frequency of carriage of weapons by visitors (especially in a military environment when all personnel are likely to be carrying weapons). There are specific circumstances where weapons may be overtly or covertly carried inside a medical facility. These should be codified as rules/procedures. All individuals carrying weapons in a medical facility are to be trained and authorised to do so with oversight by the senior leadership.

STEP 4 – DECIDE

- **What is your decision**?
- **Why** (can you justify it)?

Weapons should not be routinely allowed into the clinical areas of a military medical facility.

Rules/procedures should be put in place for specific individual circumstances if this principle has to be broken.

Further issues for consideration:

- How might local armed actors be persuaded not to enter medical facilities with weapons?
- What arrangements should be in place if visitors are expected to leave their weapons outside?
- What security activities inside medical facilities are specifically excluded under IHL – see further reading?
- What arrangements are in place in civilian hospitals for the security/protection of patients at high risk of being attacked or attacking staff? Consider how this applies within prison medical facilities

NOTES

1. The ICRC hosts a database of IHL and associated commentaries, available at https://ihl-databases.icrc.org/en.

2. Examples are as follows: US Army Values – https://www.army.mil/values/, British Army Values and Standards – https://www.army.mod.uk/who-we-are/our-people/a-soldiers-values-and-standards/, Royal Air Force – https://recruitment.raf.mod.uk/recruitment/media/3897/20200703-raf_ap1_2019_rev_3_page_spreads.pdf, Royal Navy – https://www.royalnavy.mod.uk/organisation/our-people/our-values. Australian Defence Force – https://www.defence.gov.au/about/who-we-are/values-behaviours.

3. WMA International Code of Medical Ethics – https://www.wma.net/policies-post/wma-international-code-of-medical-ethics/, World Health Organization Global Health Ethics – https://www.who.int/health-topics/ethics-and-health#tab=tab_1, United Nations Office for Human Rights – https://www.ohchr.org/en/instruments-mechanisms/instruments/principles-medical-ethics-relevant-role-health-personnel, and the International Council of Nurses – https://www.icn.ch/resources/publications-and-reports/icn-code-ethics-nurses.

4. State signatories are those states that express their consent to be bound by a treaty by signing the treaty without the need for ratification, acceptance or approval.

5. Sometimes referred to as 'medical rules of engagement', which can be confused with rules of engagement referring to the legal use of military force.

REFERENCES

1. United Nations Charter. Chapter VII: Action with Respect to Threats to the Peace, Breaches of the Peace, and Acts of Aggression. Article 51. https://www.un.org/en/about-us/un-charter/chapter-7.

2. Beauchamp, T.L. (2013). *Principles of Biomedical Ethics*, 7e (ed. J.F. Childress). New York: Oxford University Press.

3. Wilson, C.B. (2022). Dual loyalty/military medicine. *World Medical Journal* 70: 4–7. https://www.wma.net/wp-content/uploads/2022/11/WMJ_2022_03_final-1.pdf.

4. ICRC (2021). Protecting Healthcare: Guidance for the Armed Forces. https://healthcareindanger.org/wp-content/uploads/2021/03/4504_002-ebook.pdf.

5. Litz, B.T., Stein, N., Delaney, E. et al. (2009). Moral injury and moral repair in war veterans: a preliminary model and intervention strategy. *Clinical Psychology Review* 29 (8): 695–706. https://doi.org/10.1016/j.cpr.2009.07.003. Epub 2009 Jul 29. PMID: 19683376.

6. Beardmore, C., Bricknell, M., Kelly, J., and Lough, F. (2024). Commentary – a military health care ethics framework. *Military Medicine* https://doi.org/10.1093/milmed/usae351.

CHAPTER 7

Global Health Security

Ben Wakefield[1] and Martin Bricknell[2]

[1] *Johns Hopkins Center for Health Security, Baltimore, USA*
[2] *Centre for Conflict and Health Security, King's College London, London, UK*

Abstract

The aim of this chapter is to analyse the term 'global health security' and how this has placed health within the security agenda. The chapter opens by reviewing the development of the term global health security (GHS) and other phrases that have securitised health threats. It will then examine the general policies and processes needed to prevent, detect and respond to emerging health threats that have the potential to have global impact. The key health threats of pandemics (e.g. H5N1 influenza), proliferation of chemical, biological, radiological and nuclear (CBRN) weapons, and antimicrobial resistance (AMR) will then be summarised. The chapter will close by discussing the risks of securitisation of global health.

Keywords: health security, anti-microbial resistance, pandemic, surveillance, CBRN, non-proliferation

---

KEY LEARNING OUTCOMES

By studying this chapter, the reader will be able to:

- Describe the concept of global health security (GHS).
- Consider the policies and processes required to prevent, detect and respond to emerging health threats

---

Handbook of Global Health, Security, and War, First Edition. Edited by Martin Bricknell and Richard Sullivan.
© 2025 John Wiley & Sons Ltd. Published 2025 by John Wiley & Sons Ltd.

> - Investigate the key threats such as pandemic influenza, the proliferation of chemical, biological, radiological, and nuclear (CBRN) weapons, and antimicrobial resistance (AMR)
> - Consider the risks associated with the securitisation of global health

WHAT IS GLOBAL HEALTH SECURITY?

Global health as a dimension of public health was introduced in Chapter 1. Wider concepts in security were discussed in Chapter 2, which included a short overview of the concept of **global health security** (GHS) as a tool to place threats to health within the security agenda. This chapter will explore concepts that underpin the current framing of GHS including critiques that suggest that securitisation of health carries the risk of realist behaviours by states, which may undermine the liberalist approach to health as the ultimate, apolitical public good.

There is no universal definition of GHS, but it can broadly be defined as the activities required to prevent, detect and respond to infectious disease threats globally, whether they occur naturally, accidentally, or deliberately. Health security is a relatively new concept with an exponential rise in academic publications that mention 'health' and 'security' in the title or abstract from 1980 to 2022 [1]. United Nations Security Council (UNSC) Resolution 1308 of 2000 was the first time that a health issue, the HIV/AIDS pandemic, had been categorised as a potential risk to global stability and security. The Anthrax letters episode of autumn 2001 that killed 5 people and infected a further 17 people in the United States put bioterrorism into the crucible of the US Global War on Terror. Subsequently, the security discourse abruptly shifted from a unipolar state-based perception of security to a multi-dimensional perception of risk from threat actors that includes state adversaries, ideological terrorists, and transnational criminals, with the potential to use weapons of mass destruction (WMD) alongside conventional weapons. However, it should be noted that non-state actors have never successfully developed and deployed chemical, biological, radiological and nuclear (CBRN) agents on a large scale.

The Global Health Security Initiative was launched in November 2001 as an informal partnership of nine countries to strengthen public health preparedness and response to the threat of international CBRN terrorism (pandemic influenza was added in 2002). The 2005 revision to International Health Regulations (IHR) included the release of CBRN weapons alongside infectious disease as potential reasons for the Director General of the World Health Organization (WHO) to declare a Public Health Emergency of International Concern (PHEIC). McInnes and Lee showed how transnational infectious diseases (e.g. HIV/AIDS) and the emergence of drug-resistant infectious diseases (e.g. tuberculosis and the potential for biological agents to be used as terrorist weapons) became part of the security and foreign policy dialogue in the early 2000s [2].

The 2014 outbreak of Ebola in West Africa was the first health emergency in which international military forces were an integral part of the global assistance efforts to the three affected countries of Sierra Leone, Guinea, and Liberia. This outbreak further strengthened the linkage between threats to health and risks to national and global security, widened criticisms of the relative impotence of the WHO, and emphasised the need for supranational authority over sovereign states to challenge the vested interests of powerful states in the management of global health emergencies [3]. Please undertake Learning Activity 7.1 to examine the legacy of the Ebola crisis in more detail.

Learning Activity 7.1   The Ebola Crisis 2014

Watch the YouTube Video: Ebola Outbreak 360° | FRONTLINE – https://www.youtube.com/watch?v=G93XJCVr8vk

Read: Heymann, D.L., Chen, L., Takemi, K. et al. (2015). Global health security: the wider lessons from the West African Ebola virus disease epidemic. *The Lancet.* 385 (9980): 1884–1901. doi: 10.1016/S0140-6736(15)60858-3. PMID: 25987157; PMCID: PMC5856330.

- Why was the Ebola outbreak in West Africa a Public Health Emergency of International Concern?
- How did the international community mobilise to support outbreak control in the affected West African countries?
- What measures did unaffected countries take to protect their populations' health?
- What were the lessons from this health crisis for the protection of global health?

Suggested answers are at the end of the chapter.

The term 'global health security' became more prominent in both health and security debates after the Ebola crisis. The Global Health Security Agenda (GHSA) was launched by the US Centre for Disease Control in 2014 as a group of 69 countries, international and non-government organisations, and private sector companies to collectively strengthen the global ability to prevent, detect, and respond to infectious disease threats. The Global Health Security Index is an international assessment of GHS capabilities in 195 countries prepared by the Johns Hopkins Center for Health Security. The first analysis was published in 2019 with an update in 2021. Notably, a high GHS index score did not correlate with a lower number of COVID-19 cases or deaths, though it was associated with vaccination coverage [4].

As discussed in Chapter 2, threats to health became acknowledged as threats to security during the 2010s. The UK Strategic Defence and Security Review of 2010 included civil emergencies for the first time in the form of natural hazards or accidents (including influenza pandemics) as a Tier 1 risk, and an attack on the United Kingdom or its Overseas Territories by another state or proxy using chemical, biological, radiological or nuclear (CBRN) weapons as Tier 2 priority [5]. The inclusion of health threats and the linkage to CBRN weapons have been a feature of subsequent

UK security reviews, including the 2023 UK Biological Security Strategy [6], and are replicated in other nations' security policies. The United States first published a National Biodefense Strategy in 2018 [7], and subsequently published an updated strategy in 2022 [8], as well as Global Health Security Strategies in 2019 [9] and 2024 [10]. These documents cover both domestic preparedness for health emergencies and international collaboration to help other countries develop their own health security capabilities.

COMPONENTS OF GHS AND ONE HEALTH

The WHO defines global public health security as

> *The activities required, both proactive and reactive, to minimize the danger and impact of acute public health events that endanger people's health across geographical regions and international boundaries* [11].

The list of health hazards includes infectious disease outbreaks, conflicts, natural disasters, chemical or radio-nuclear spills, and water and food contamination. The World Health Assembly (WHA) has a long history of encouraging member states to strengthen their public health system response to health emergencies. WHA Resolution 64 of 2011 urged member states to strengthen disaster risk reduction, emergency preparedness and response within their health systems [12].

It has been increasingly recognised that outbreaks of infectious disease (or other health hazards) in plants and animals can also impact human health, either by mutation into phytonotic (plant-to-human transmission – rare) or zoonotic (animal-to-human transmission – common) diseases that can affect humans or by their impact on food, water, and general environment. This has been described as 'One Health', defined as follows:

> *an integrated, unifying approach that aims to sustainably balance and optimize the health of people, animals, and ecosystems* [13].

The One Health approach aims to address the full spectrum of activities to mitigate health threats from prevention, health improvement, and health promotion to the detection, preparedness, response, and recovery from health crises. At the global level, this guides collaboration between the UN Food and Agriculture Organization, the World Organization for Animal Health, the United Nations Environment Programme, and the WHO. At the national level, governments have begun to include a One Health approach as an integral part of their preparedness and response planning. For example, both the UK Biological Security Strategy and the US National Biodefense Strategy referenced in Section 1 have a One Health approach at their core. Figure 7.1 shows the interrelationships for One Health.

One health promotes a sustainable and healthy future through collaboration, communication, coordination ad capacity building

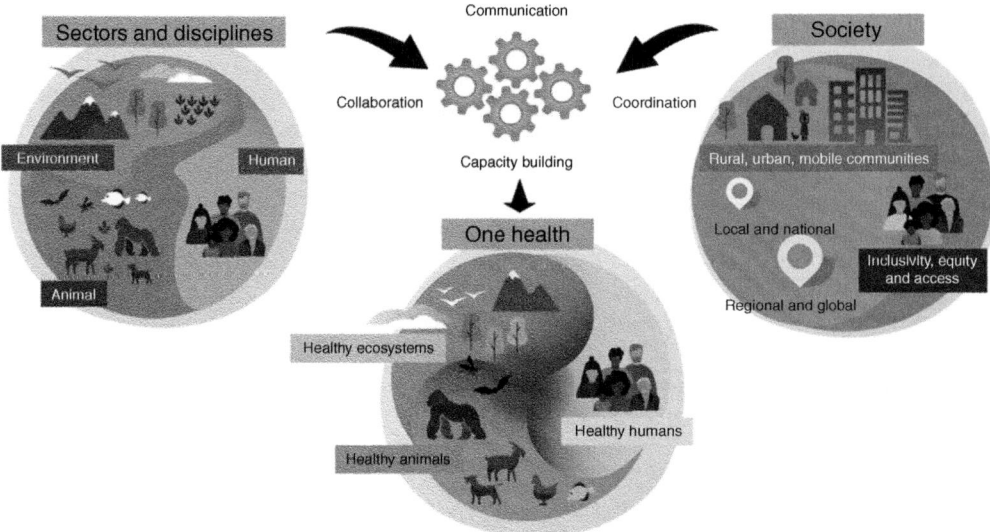

SOURCE: FAO, UNEP, WHO, and WOAH. 2022. One Health Joint Plan of Action (2022–2026). Working together for the health of humans, animals, plants and the environment. Rome. https://doi.org/10.4060/cc2289en

FIGURE 7.1   Interrelationships for One Health.

PANDEMICS

There is no universally agreed definition of a pandemic. It can be considered as simultaneous outbreaks of the same infectious disease occurring worldwide or over a very wide area, crossing international boundaries, and infecting a large number of people, animals or plants. There is no definition of a pandemic in the IHR 2005, and instead, actions (such as the release of emergency funds) are linked to the declaration of a PHEIC. This is defined as follows:

> *An extraordinary event which is determined to constitute a public health risk to other States through the international spread of disease and to potentially require a coordinated international response* [14].

According to the WHO, this definition of a PHEIC implies a situation that is:

- serious, sudden, unusual or unexpected;
- carries implications for public health beyond the affected state's national border and
- may require immediate international action [15].

It therefore follows that not all PHEICs are necessarily pandemics (such as the 2014–2016 Ebola outbreak), and an outbreak may be a pandemic before it is categorised as a PHEIC.

Within the IHR 2005, Member States of the World Health Assembly are required to have the ability to detect, assess and report, and respond to public health risks and emergencies. As part of this, member states may voluntarily seek a Joint External Evaluation (JEE) of their status and progress in developing capacity to prevent, detect and rapidly respond to public health threats [16]. The JEE is structured around the following high-level headings:

1. Prevent
2. Detect
3. Respond, and
4. Others (points of entry, chemical events and radiation emergencies).

The 69 members of the GHSA committed to support each other to work towards the performance goals within the JEE framework. This international cooperation is often contained within a county's Global Health Security Strategy or equivalent document. Chapter 8 will discuss the response to health crises at the health system level. A scoping review of international programmes to support low- and middle-income countries (LMICs) to strengthen their public health capabilities identified five key factors for the effectiveness of such health systems strengthening activities. These were as follows:

1. Training and skills development for the public health workforce
2. Sustainable financial investment for people, money and infrastructure
3. Integration of GHS capacity building within wider health systems strengthening and universal health coverage
4. Multi-sectoral coordination using 'all-hazards' and One Health approaches
5. Effective and equitable partnership working [17].

The report of the Lancet Commission on synergies between three themes of universal health coverage, health security, and health promotion provides an analysis of the risks and opportunities associated with international development assistance for health programmes [18]. There are very clear synergies across these themes, but there is a risk that emphasis on each individual theme can cause fragmentation of effort unless there is an explicit effort to coordinate across multiple bilateral and multilateral donor programmes.

The COVID-19 crisis exemplified the logic of a pandemic being a threat to multiple dimensions of national security. Observations for GHS from the COVID-19 crisis are contained in Learning Activities within Chapters 10 and 15 of this book. Since the end of the pandemic, the WHO and its Member States have been working on negotiating a new pandemic treaty and an update to the IHR 2005. The behaviours of stakeholders in these negotiations are discussed through an International Relations lens in Chapter 16. Chapter 10 on War, Communicable Disease and Health Security will cover the principles for the management of an outbreak of infectious disease at local, national, and international levels.

CBRN WEAPONS

Chapter 5 provided an overview of the biomedical understanding of the impact of CBRN weapons on the human body and introduced the international treaties and conventions which aspire to reduce the risk of accidental and deliberate release of these agents by states or other armed actors. The GHS approach to the threats from a pandemic could be considered as a neutral, apolitical activity focussed on health as a public good, whereas the GHS approach towards reducing risks from the accidental or deliberate release of CBRN weapons is more grounded in the 'hard' security perspective that led to the founding of the Global Health Security Initiative. As discussed in the section 'Pandemics' of this chapter, the JEE framework includes a detailed assessment of biological laboratory capabilities and the response to chemical and radiological events.

The Global Health Security Initiative emerged from the US-led CBRN Cooperative Threat Reduction Program initiated by the Nunn-Lugar Act in 1991 (also known as the Soviet Threat Reduction Act) after the fall of the Soviet Union. This programme attempted to re-purpose ex-Soviet CBRN research capabilities by reducing laboratory stockpiles of weapons-grade research material, providing alternative investment to encourage scientists to undertake non-military research, and to establish legal and ethical regimes for chemical and biological research.

Recent developments in biomedical sciences research, both scientific (e.g. genetic engineering) and computational (e.g. artificial intelligence), are fundamentally 'dual use'. Whilst these can be developed and used for peaceful purposes, they may also increase the technical possibilities for the development of advanced chemical and biological weapons that could be both more lethal and more targeted than currently recognised agents. These technologies are becoming more widespread and accessible, which may also increase the risk of use by non-state actors. However, the peaceful applications of these technologies may also reduce the impact of malicious use, by facilitating rapid advancements in the development of effective or novel medical counter-measures or surveillance and detection methods. This could produce a 'deterrence-by-denial' effect, where actors are dissuaded from using biological or chemical weapons as their impact might be easily countered or mitigated, rendering their effort unsuccessful.

Chapter 5 introduced the Biological and Toxin Weapons Convention (BTWC or BWC), which prohibits the development, production, acquisition, transfer, stockpiling and use of biological and toxin weapons [19]. The Chemical Weapons Convention prohibits the development, production, stockpiling and use of chemical weapons, mandates their destruction, and is overseen by the Organisation for the Prohibition of Chemical Weapons (OPCW) [20]. Further to this, UN Security Council Resolution 1540 (2004) requires that:

All States shall refrain from providing any form of support to non-State actors that attempt to develop, acquire, manufacture, possess, transport, transfer or use nuclear, chemical or biological weapons and their means of delivery, in particular for terrorist purposes [21].

The GHS approach to chemical and biological weapons is founded upon widening and strengthening these treaties and conventions (among others), and the international norms against the use of biological weapons (BW) and chemical weapons (CW) that they help to uphold, underpinned by the monitoring and detection of research and development programmes that are acting outside these international agreements. The demonstrated use of chemical weapons in Syria by the Assad regime and in targeted assassinations in the United Kingdom and elsewhere by the Russian Federation, as well as the malicious disinformation efforts surrounding these incidents, have undermined the international norms against the use of chemical weapons.

Under the BWC, states are encouraged to exchange confidence-building measures such as sharing current biodefence activities, disease outbreaks, key life sciences publications, national biosecurity legislation and other measures, and high-risk pathogen research and vaccine production facilities [22]. Unfortunately, the increasing tension within the international system is making these exchanges more difficult. Unlike the chemical weapons convention (CWC), the BWC has no verification or investigation mechanism. Studies into the origin of the COVID-19 virus demonstrated the difficulties with investigation and attribution of biological events [23]. There have been suggestions that the military approach to intelligence could be applied to health security threats and that classified intelligence collection methods should also be used to capture information about health threats in and from other states [24].

ANTIMICROBIAL RESISTANCE

The development of penicillin and other antibiotics has transformed modern medicine. Antimicrobial resistance (AMR) is the emergence of organisms that are resistant to drugs that are used to prevent or treat infections. This is increasing and represents one of the greatest risks to public health and health security with estimates of up to 4.95 million deaths in 2019 and up to 10 million additional deaths by 2050 attributable to drug resistance [25]. Whilst the focus of concern is on antibiotic-resistant bacteria that cause human infections, antibiotic-resistant bacteria and other organisms (viruses, fungi) can also cause infections in animals and plants. Intervention strategies rely on basic infection prevention and control within healthcare settings, vaccination as an alternative to antibiotic treatment, controlling the use of antibiotics in animal husbandry and human health, and investing in research for new antibiotics. In 2024, the United Nations General Assembly reaffirmed the commitment of its members to address AMR [26].

Despite AMR appearing as a security issue in policy documents, it could be argued that there is a lack of urgency in addressing this element of GHS compared to public health emergencies that rapidly affect health systems and the global economy. AMR is a One Health issue that requires a multisectoral global response that is applicable to all countries. This requires a health system approach covering prevention, surveillance and monitoring, changes in expectations and use of antibiotics, and clear regulation and advice on the appropriate use of antimicrobials. High-income countries (HICs) can be the catalyst for developing new drugs but must avoid creating unmanageable financial burdens on LMICs in stewardship of antibiotic use [27]. Please undertake the Case Study in Learning Activity 7.2 to examine the challenge with managing AMR during war.

Learning Activity 7.2   Case Study – Antimicrobial Resistance (AMR) and War

Read:

Pallett, S.J., Boyd, S.E., O'Shea, M.K. et al. (2023). The contribution of human conflict to the development of antimicrobial resistance. *Communications Medicine* 3 (1): 153. https://doi.org/10.1038/s43856-023-00386-7.

Consider the following questions:

- Why might war be a crucible for AMR?
- How might the risks of AMR be mitigated during war?
- What additional constraints would a conflict environment place on countering the risks of AMR?

Suggested answers are at the end of the chapter.

RISKS FROM SECURITISING HEALTH

Securitisation theory in international relations can be viewed as a process that justifies the use of security instruments to manage an 'existential threat', escalating what might be a low-priority issue to a high-priority issue by using a national security framing to move the issue beyond politics. This can convince a target audience that 'emergency measures' which control populations and restrict their rights are justified to protect the national interest.

Some framing of GHS strategies from Global North or HICs can be perceived as colonialist, as they might frame the issue as protecting their citizens from threats that are coming from the Global South or LMICs that need to be controlled and managed, rather than a global threat to be tackled through international cooperation [28]. Thus, GHS may become an instrument of security and foreign policy rather than international development [2]. Measures taken by HICs during health emergencies, such as border closures, restriction of movement of people and goods, and surveillance, can have a relatively more severe impact on LMICs. The IHR 2005 warns against the negative impacts of restrictions on travel and trade during an outbreak.

Technical assistance such as laboratory capacity building can be implemented as an equitable partnership, but it can also be used in an extractive way. This might be as an intelligence-gathering exercise to collect biological samples from around the world for national research or to exclude the host country from the scientific and economic benefits of these samples.

The use of armed forces as part of a global response to outbreaks of infectious disease also provides a highly public message of securitisation and depending on the social, political and cultural context can have a negative impact on the response or even risk harm to health workers. This language of 'security against' may also be applied to other health threats such as obesity and drug misuse. This contrasts with a language of universality and equity that sees health as a public good in which the wealthy have a duty to support the less well-off [29].

LOOKING FORWARD

This chapter has provided a short overview to GHS and how the mitigation of health threats can be an element of national security policy. It specifically considered pandemics, CBRN weapons, and AMR as threats that can be commonly included within national security risk assessments. The chapter closed by discussing some risks associated with 'securitisation' of health. This chapter completes Part 1 of the book on perspectives on global health and security. Part 2 will deconstruct each component of the health system response to the challenges of insecurity and war.

SOURCES AND RESOURCES

Suggested Internet search terms are as follows: 'global health security', 'health security', 'antimicrobial resistance', 'threat reduction programme', 'CBRN', 'WMD', and 'Dual-use Research'.

Suggested websites for further information are as follows:

WHO Webpages:

- Antimicrobial resistance, available at `https://www.who.int/health-topics/antimicrobial-resistance`
- Biological Weapons, available at `https://www.who.int/health-topics/biological-weapons#tab=tab_1`
- Health security, available at `https://www.who.int/health-topics/health-security#tab=tab_1`
- Strengthening the global health-security interface, available at `https://www.who.int/activities/strengthening-the-global-health-security-interface`

United Nations Office for Disarmament Affairs (UNODA), available at `https://disarmament.unoda.org/wmd/`. UNODA supports specialised agencies of the UN and other intergovernmental organisations in the area of disarmament and non-proliferation of WMD (nuclear, chemical and biological weapons).

GHSA, available at `https://globalhealthsecurityagenda.org/`. A global effort to strengthen the world's ability to prevent, detect, and respond to infectious disease threats.

Global Health Security Initiative (GHSI), available at `http://ghsi.ca/`. An informal, international partnership among like-minded countries and organisations to strengthen public health preparedness and response globally to threats of chemical, biological, and radio-nuclear terrorism (CBRN), as well as pandemic influenza.

The Global Health Security Index (GHSI), available at `https://ghsindex.org/`. This measures the capacities of 195 countries to prepare for epidemics and pandemics. The most recent assessment is dated 2021.

Walsh, P.F. (Ed.). (2024). *Health Security Intelligence: Managing Emerging Threats and Risks in a Post-Covid World* (1st ed.). Routledge. Available at `https://doi.org/10.4324/9781003335511`.

Learning Activity 7.1   The Ebola Crisis 2014 – Suggested Answers

- **Why was the Ebola 2014 outbreak in West Africa a Public Health Emergency of International Concern?** *The WHO classified the 2014 Ebola outbreak a PHEIC because of the continuing transmission of Ebola in West African communities and health facilities, the high case fatality rate of Ebola virus disease (EVD), and the weak health services of Guinea, Liberia, Sierra Leone, Nigeria, and other neighbouring countries at risk for infection. This declaration imposed obligations on the affected countries and the whole international community* [30].

- **How did the international community mobilise to support outbreak control in the affected West African countries?** *They deployed civilian agencies and military personnel to augment the capacity of affected countries to manage the outbreak. They help to set up reporting and surveillance systems, treatment centres, procedures and capacity for safe burials, and social mobilisation to ensure public support for the draconian control measures.*

- **What measures did unaffected countries take to protect their populations' health?** *Imposed health screening for all travellers from the affected region, banned international travel for cases and travellers with a raised body temperature, created biological containment pods for aeromedical evacuation of expatriates from the affected area and reinforced existing systems for the containment and treatment of potential cases arising locally.*

- **What were the lessons from this health crisis for the protection of global health?** *Reinforced the principles of health security: an empowered and resourced WHO; national capacity for detection, identification, and control of outbreaks of infectious diseases; the need for national and global stockpiles of key commodities required to control an outbreak of disease (e.g. personal protective equipment (PPE) and vaccines); capacity for rapid mobilisation of the scientific community and commercial biosciences industries to develop testing kits and vaccinations; generation of an emergency response fund; and removal of regulatory and trade barriers that inhibit knowledge transfer from the Global North to the South.*

Learning Activity 7.2   Case Study – Antimicrobial Resistance (AMR) and War – Suggested Answers

Consider the following questions:

- **Why might war be a crucible for AMR?**

    War is an epidemic of injuries.

    War wounds tend to be infected, and treatment delayed.

    War wounds tend to be larger and more difficult to clean and close than other traumatic wounds.

    War injuries tend to be treated in several different medical units, increasing the risk of transfer of AMR organisms between facilities.

    War injuries tend to receive multiple 'cocktails' of antibiotics.

    War destroys the natural and man-made environment creating unsafe and unsanitary conditions for medical treatment, heightening the risk of infection. The destruction caused by war can contaminate the environment with heavy metals and chemicals, which increases the risk of/stimulates AMR.

- **How might the risks of AMR be mitigated during war?**

    Recognition of a potential problem.

    Detailed attention to infection prevention and control procedures when receiving patients with longstanding wounds.

    Establishment of a microbiological surveillance system.

    Establishment of an antibiotic use policy to reduce the use of broad-spectrum, multi-drug 'cocktails'.

    Financial, technical and logistic assistance to countries at war to support the implementation of AMR national action plans.

- **What additional constraints would a conflict environment place on countering the risks of AMR?**

    The destructive and contaminating elements of war discussed in question 1 are difficult to avoid.

    Soldiers and field medics can only carry a finite amount of equipment and therefore pragmatic choices must be made in terms of what antibiotics are most effective.

REFERENCES

1. McCoy, D., Roberts, S., Daoudi, S., and Kennedy, J. (2023). Global health security and the health-security nexus: principles, politics and praxis. *BMJ Global Health.* 8 (9): e013067. https://doi.org/10.1136/bmjgh-2023-013067.

2. McInnes, C. and Lee, K. (2006). Health, security and foreign policy. *Review of International Studies.* 32 (1): 5–23. https://doi.org/10.1017/S0260210506006905.

3. Gostin, L.O. (2016). Global health security after Ebola: four global commissions. *The Milbank Quarterly.* 94 (1): 34–38. https://doi.org/10.1111/1468-0009.12176.

4. Alhassan, R.K., Nketiah-Amponsah, E., Afaya, A. et al. (2023). Global Health Security Index not a proven surrogate for health systems capacity to respond to pandemics: The case of COVID-19. *Journal of Infection and Public Health* 16 (2): 196–205. https://doi.org/10.1016/j.jiph.2022.12.011. Epub 2022 Dec 21. PMID: 36584636; PMCID: PMC9769026.

5. Cabinet Office (2010). Securing Britain in an Age of Uncertainty: The Strategic Defence and Security Review. CM7948. https://www.gov.uk/government/publications/the-strategic-defence-and-security-review-securing-britain-in-an-age-of-uncertainty.

6. HM Government (2023). UK Biological Security Strategy. https://assets.publishing.service.gov.uk/media/64c0ded51e10bf000e17ceba/UK_Biological_Security_Strategy.pdf.

7. National Biodefense Strategy (2018) The White House. https://trumpwhitehouse.archives.gov/wp-content/uploads/2018/09/National-Biodefense-Strategy.pdf.

8. National Biodefense Strategy and Implementation Plan (2022). The White House. https://www.whitehouse.gov/wp-content/uploads/2022/10/National-Biodefense-Strategy-and-Implementation-Plan-Final.pdf.

9. United States Government Global Health Security Strategy (2019). The White House. https://trumpwhitehouse.archives.gov/wp-content/uploads/2019/05/GHSS.pdf.

10. U.S. Government Global Health Security Strategy (2024). The White House. https://www.whitehouse.gov/wp-content/uploads/2024/04/Global-Health-Security-Strategy-2024-1.pdf.

11. World Health Organisation. Health Security. Geneva: World Health Organisation. https://www.who.int/health-topics/health-security#tab=tab_1.

12. World Health Assembly, 64 (2011). Strengthening national health emergency and disaster management capacities and resilience of health systems. World Health Organization. https://iris.who.int/handle/10665/3566.

13. One Health High-Level Expert Panel (OHHLEP), Adisasmito, W.B., Almuhairi, S. et al. (2022). One Health: A new definition for a sustainable and healthy future. *PLoS Pathogens* 18 (6): e1010537. https://doi.org/10.1371/journal.ppat.101.

14. International Health Regulations (2005). WHO. https://www.who.int/publications/i/item/9789241580496.

15. WHO Newsroom. Emergencies: International health regulations and emergency committees. https://www.who.int/news-room/questions-and-answers/item/emergencies-international-health-regulations-and-emergency-committees.

16. World Health Organization (2022). *Joint External Evaluation Tool: International Health Regulations (2005)*, 3e. Geneva: World Health Organization Licence: CC BY-NC-SA 3.0 IGO. https://www.who.int/publications/i/item/9789240051980.

17. Doble, A., Sheridan, Z., Razavi, A. et al. (2023). The role of international support programmes in global health security capacity building: a scoping review. *PLOS*

Global Public Health 3 (4): e0001763. https://doi.org/10.1371/journal. pgph.0001763.

18. Agyepong, I., Spicer, N., Ooms, G. et al. (2023). Lancet Commission on synergies between universal health coverage, health security, and health promotion. *The Lancet* 401 (10392): 1964–2012. https://doi.org/10.1016/S0140-6736(22)01930-4.

19. UNODA. Biological Weapons Convention. https://disarmament.unoda.org/ biological-weapons/.

20. OPCW. Chemical Weapons Convention. https://www.opcw.org/chemical-weapons-convention.

21. UNODA. UN Security Council Resolution 1540. https://disarmament.unoda. org/wmd/sc1540/.

22. Edwards, B., Novossiolova, T., Crowley, M. et al. (2022). Meeting the challenges of chemical and biological weapons: strengthening the chemical and biological disarmament and non-proliferation regimes. *Frontiers in Political Science* 4: 805426. https:// doi.org/10.3389/fpos.2022.805426.

23. Yassif, J.M., Korol, S., and Kane, A. (2023). Guarding against catastrophic biological risks: preventing state biological weapon development and use by shaping intentions. *Health Security.* 21 (4): 258–265. https://doi.org/10.1089/hs.2022.0145.

24. Bowsher, G. Building better health security intelligence strategies post-COVID-19. In: *Health Security Intelligence* (ed. P.F. Walsh), 79–97. Routledge: https:// www.taylorfrancis.com/reader/read-online/4d7b9e8d-0e59-477c-b3e7-472579e4b481/chapter/pdf?context=ubx.

25. Murray, C.J., Ikuta, K.S., Sharara, F. et al. (2022). Global burden of bacterial antimicrobial resistance in 2019: a systematic analysis. *The Lancet.* 399 (10325): 629–655. https://doi.org/10.1016/S0140-6736(21)02724-0.

26. UN General Assembly (2024). Political Declaration of the High-level Meeting on Antimicrobial Resistance. https://www.un.org/pga/wp-content/uploads/ sites/108/2024/09/FINAL-Text-AMR-to-PGA.pdf.

27. Cars, O., Chandy, S.J., Mpundu, M. et al. (2021). Resetting the agenda for antibiotic resistance through a health systems perspective. *The Lancet Global Health* 9 (7): e1022–e1027. https://doi.org/10.1016/S2214-109X(21)00163-7.

28. Rushton, S. (2011). Global Health Security: Security for whom? Security from what? *Political Studies* 59 (4): 779–796. https://doi.org/10.1111/j.1467-9248.2011.00919.x.

29. Holst, J. and van de Pas, R. (2023). The biomedical securitization of global health. *Global Health* 19: 15. https://doi.org/10.1186/s12992-023-00915-y.

30. Briand, S., Bertherat, E., Cox, P. et al. (2014). The international Ebola emergency. *New England Journal of Medicine.* 371 (13): 1180–1183. https://doi.org/10.1056/ NEJMp1409858.

PART 2

HEALTH SERVICES AND CONFLICT

This second part examines how the different clinical services within a health system respond to the impact of conflict and other health emergencies on the health of affected populations. The topics selected are those from the chapter on Health within the Sphere Handbook.

Chapter 8 looks at the response of a whole health system to a crisis including the international humanitarian system. This chapter will also look at the Humanitarian Charter. Chapter 9 considers the care of physical trauma patients and the concept of a chain or pathway of care. Chapter 10 discusses the impact of war on communicable disease and also provides a link back to Chapter 7 on Global Health Security. Chapter 11 describes the impact of war on maternal and child health. Chapter 12 covers war, noncommunicable disease, and palliative care. The final chapter, Chapter 13, in this section examines war and mental health. Figure P2.1 shows a news image of casualties from Israeli attacks on Gaza in October 2023 arriving at a Palestinian hospital. This graphic image reflects the reality of human suffering in war.

After completing this section, the reader will be able to

- Describe how health services respond to insecurity or crisis.
- Describe the provision of clinical services to care for physical trauma patients in war.
- Describe the relationships between war, communicable disease, and global health security.
- Describe how war affects maternal and child health and the essential clinical services needed to meet the needs of these patients.

Handbook of Global Health, Security, and War, First Edition. Edited by Martin Bricknell and Richard Sullivan.
© 2025 John Wiley & Sons Ltd. Published 2025 by John Wiley & Sons Ltd.

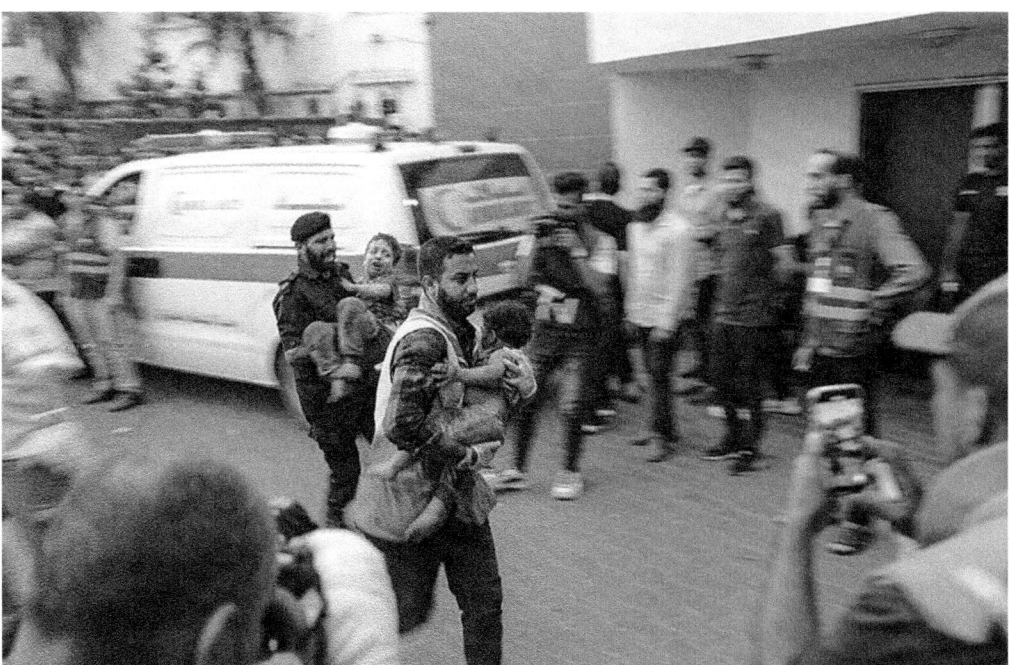

FIGURE P2.1 Medics transported an injured Palestinian child into Al-Shifa Hospital in Gaza City following an Israeli airstrike on 11 October 2023. *Source*: Palestinian News & Information Agency (WAFA) / CC BY-SA 3.0 / https://commons.wikimedia.org/wiki/File:Damage_in_Gaza_Strip_during_the_October_2023_-_38.jpg / last accessed February 07, 2025.

- Describe the provision of clinical services to care for non-communicable disease patients and how to provide palliative care during war.
- Describe the impact of conflict on mental health services and clinical services for individuals and communities.

CHAPTER 8

Health Systems Response to Crises

Adarsh Tiwathia[1] and Martin Bricknell[2]

[1] *Former Deputy Director of the Division of Healthcare Management and Occupational Safety and Health, United Nations, New York, NY, USA*
[2] *Centre for Conflict and Health Security, King's College London, UK*

Abstract

The aim of this chapter is to understand how health systems respond to insecurity or crises. In conflict situations, healthcare providers tend to focus on the provision of life-saving health services with less focus on a health system approach. Whilst life-saving health services should always be at the core of any health intervention in conflict situations, some efforts should be paid to sustaining health interventions through investing in strengthening health systems. This chapter builds upon the discussions from Chapter 1 on health systems and Chapter 3 on the impact of war on health. It will describe the international humanitarian system and the role of international agencies (IAs) and international non-government organisations (iNGOs) in supporting local communities. Following the approach of the health chapter in the Sphere Handbook, this chapter will then consider the key standards for a health system covering access, competence of health professionals, provision of medicines and medical devices, and monitoring of quality and outcomes.

Keywords: emergency planning, humanitarian principles, cluster system, NGOs

Handbook of Global Health, Security, and War, First Edition. Edited by Martin Bricknell and Richard Sullivan.

KEY LEARNING OUTCOMES

By studying this chapter, the reader will be able to:

- Describe the essential elements of health systems in their response to conflict and crises
- Describe the UN cluster system
- Summarise the Sphere Project
- List some international non-government organisations (iNGOs) that provide health services
- Recognise attacks on healthcare
- Research the practical aspects of health systems response in Syria as a result of the civil war

---

NATIONAL RESPONSE TO EMERGENCIES

Unfortunately, as outlined in Chapter 2, conflict and war are an inherent dimension of societal behaviours both internally and externally within states. Endemic political tension underpins the intractable conflicts in the sub-Saharan countries of Africa, Haiti, Libya, Yemen, the wider Middle East, Myanmar, and more recently the Eastern European countries bordering Russia. Beyond conflict, natural disasters (earthquakes, extreme weather, outbreaks of infectious disease) can also cause such human suffering that a national, regional and global emergency humanitarian response may be required.

Chapter 1 introduced some concepts in emergency planning for the health system response to a major incident or health emergency. Chapter 2 identified the importance of health systems in the response to security crises as these almost invariably have the potential to cause large numbers of casualties, either as the secondary consequence of the security threat (such as a terrorist incident) or as the primary emergency (such as an outbreak of infectious disease). Both chapters introduced the concept of **resilience** as an instrument of national power to reflect the importance of responding to and recovering from a security crisis. The resilience of the national health system is a vital element of the **critical national infrastructure** that maintains essential services for citizens during any emergency.

This chapter is based upon Section 1.1 Health Systems of the Health Chapter in the Sphere Handbook at pages 297–310. This chapter will expand this discussion by considering a range of models and frameworks for the health systems and wider governance of response to emergencies. As a starting point, please complete Learning Activity 8.1.

The international system is underpinned by the principle of sovereignty in which states, and their governments, have the primary responsibility to meet the needs of their citizens. This includes the duty to manage the response to disasters and other emergencies. The **Sendai Framework**, sponsored by the United Nations Office for Disaster Risk Reduction, is a global framework for the management of disaster risk that provides a structure for the adoption of policies, strategies and plans at

Learning Activity 8.1   ReliefWeb and WHO Emergencies Review

Copy the World Map in Figure 8.2 in the Appendix to this chapter.
Go to the ReliefWeb website at https://reliefweb.int/
Select the 'Disasters' tab.
Colour the locations of these disasters on your map.
Compare your map with the World Health Organization (WHO) list of ongoing health emergencies at https://www.who.int/emergencies/situations
Consider the following questions:

Where are the humanitarian crises today?
What are the categories of disasters that cause humanitarian emergencies?

local, national, regional and global levels to reduce disaster risk and losses in lives, livelihoods and health.[1] It has five priorities for action: improve understanding of disaster risk; strengthen disaster risk governance; invest in disaster risk reduction for resilience; enhance disaster preparedness for effective response; and 'Build Back Better' in recovery, rehabilitation and reconstruction. Disaster management can be considered as a cycle of phases of disaster management: prevention, mitigation, preparedness, response, and recovery. Many states have established a **National Disaster Management Authority** (or other agency) that co-ordinates the activities of government departments, civil society, volunteers and community-based organisations as part of a national disaster management plan.

Chapter 1 introduced the concept of a '**major medical incident**' as part of the local re-adjustment of priorities for a health system within the response to an event that has caused a large number of casualties or patients. At a system level, national health systems require inherent resilience so as to have the organisational and structural capacity to respond to a disaster. The implementation of the Sendai Framework within a health system requires the integration of **disaster risk management** into the levels of primary, secondary and tertiary healthcare, especially at the local level. Health workers need to understand **disaster risk** and apply and implement **disaster risk reduction** approaches in health work, including the promotion and delivery of training in the field of disaster medicine. Alongside the training of healthcare workers in their skills, they must also support and train community health groups in disaster risk reduction approaches within health programmes, in collaboration with other sectors such as education. As mitigation for the specific health threats from epidemic disease, it is important to implement the International Health Regulations (2005) of the WHO.[2] These approaches cross all of the building blocks for a health system described in Chapter 1, especially covering the perspectives of Public Health and Emergency Care. The WHO has characterised this planning as a Health Emergency and Disaster Risk Management (EDRM) Framework [1]. The COVID-19 pandemic of 2020–2022 was an example of a health emergency that required a massive and sustained disaster response from all elements of national and global health systems.

The acronym **EPPRR** (emergency prevention, preparedness, response and resilience) is often used to summarise the individual phases of disaster risk management. This requires five capabilities (5cs): collaborative surveillance; community protection; safe and scalable care; access to countermeasures; and emergency coordination [2]. Health emergencies can present themselves as a 'big bang' such as earthquake or disaster event, a 'rising tide' such as an evolving disease outbreak, or as a secondary impact of other security events such an outbreak of public disorder or war. A surveillance system detects and monitors both health threats and health service activity/capacity in order to identify the emergence of a health emergency. Community protection is based on establishing the community and local resilience to mitigate, respond and absorb the impact of a health emergency including the administration of vaccinations and other protective interventions. Building upon the concept of a major medical incident from Chapter 1, health systems must have the plans, people, and infrastructure to expand and re-focus resources to deliver safe and scalable urgent clinical care that covers the needs of populations affected by health emergencies. This section of the book has chapters which cover the main clinical services that may be needed to respond to the physical, psychological, and social health components of emergencies. Some health crises have specific countermeasures that are needed to mitigate the impacts on health. These include specialist diagnostics, drugs, vaccines, medical devices and medical equipment. For example, an infectious disease outbreak may necessitate new diagnostic tests, antibiotics, or vaccines; a nuclear incident may require radiological monitoring equipment, preventive administration of iodine, and specific blood tests on exposed individuals; the release of a chemical weapon may require decontamination of exposed individuals, administration of specific antidotes, and expansion of very specific clinical services (e.g. respiratory intensive care); and all health emergencies may create a surge of demand for supportive mental health services.

Emergency response plans will have a tiered level of responses with the initial surge in local resources expanding to regional or national levels depending on the intensity, scale, and duration of the crisis. Chapter 3 described the impact of war on health and health systems. This showed how war both creates a surge in demand for health services due to physical and mental trauma and also displaces services resulting in unmet need for care for chronic conditions. Furthermore, war can also affect the health workforce, damage health infrastructure, disrupt medical logistics and upset education programmes for health professionals. Whilst war is the most extreme form of health emergency, natural disasters can have many similar effects on local health services and systems. If countries are not able to manage a humanitarian emergency within their own resources, or if a state's government is not capable of providing a sufficient or equitable response, regional countries and the wider international system (often under a United Nations mandate) will mobilise resources to help to mitigate the humanitarian consequences of the crisis.

INTERNATIONAL RESPONSES TO HUMANITARIAN EMERGENCIES

The global catastrophes of the First and Second World Wars set the conditions for the creation of the United Nations as a global community of states to work together to minimise the risks of humanitarian crises and to collectively provide a response to these

TABLE 8.1   The definitions of the humanitarian principles [4].

Principle	Definition
Humanity	Human suffering must be addressed wherever it is found. The purpose of humanitarian action is to protect life and health and ensure respect for human beings
Neutrality	Humanitarian actors must not take sides in hostilities or engage in controversies of a political, racial, religious or ideological nature
Impartiality	Humanitarian action must be carried out on the basis of need alone, giving priority to the most urgent cases of distress and making no distinctions on the basis of nationality, race, gender, religious belief, class or political opinions
Operational independence	Humanitarian action must be autonomous from the political, economic, military or other objectives that any actor may hold with regard to areas where humanitarian action is being implemented

emergencies. UN General Assembly Resolution 46/182 of 1991 describes the principles and framework for humanitarian assistance and the role of the United Nations and its agencies [3]. It established the humanitarian principles of humanity, neutrality, and impartiality. This list was later increased to include 'operational independence'. These principles provide the foundation for the work of UN agencies, international non-government organisations (iNGOs), and all other stakeholders who contribute to the response to a humanitarian crisis. The definitions for each of these principles are shown in Table 8.1.

In 1992, the Department of Humanitarian Affairs was created which became the Office for the Coordination of Humanitarian Affairs (UN OCHA) in 1998. UN OCHA has five core functions of coordination, advocacy and communications, humanitarian financing, policy, and information management. UN OCHA sponsors the UN cluster system as a framework for the coordination of the response to a humanitarian emergency with a designated UN Humanitarian Coordinator delegating a UN lead agency as the sponsor for coordination of response in each domain by all stakeholders. Figure 8.1 shows the assignment of themes and lead agencies within the UN cluster system. The WHO is the designated lead for health.

The Emergency Relief Coordinator is responsible for the conduct of a multi-cluster/sector initial rapid needs assessment (MIRA) to form the basis for the strategic plan for emergency response. The WHO will conduct a health needs assessment which will identify the most immediate health problems and needs, review public health risks (e.g. disease outbreaks, malnutrition, access gaps), and map the resources that are available and the resources that are needed to deliver effective assistance. This will include an assessment of the existing health providers and infrastructure. The Health Cluster Guide published by the WHO advises how the health cluster lead agency, coordinator and partners can work together during a humanitarian crisis to achieve the aims of reducing avoidable mortality, morbidity and disability, and restoring the delivery of and equitable access to preventive and curative health care [5]. Stakeholders in the Health Cluster will include the WHO, the Ministry of Health, local health

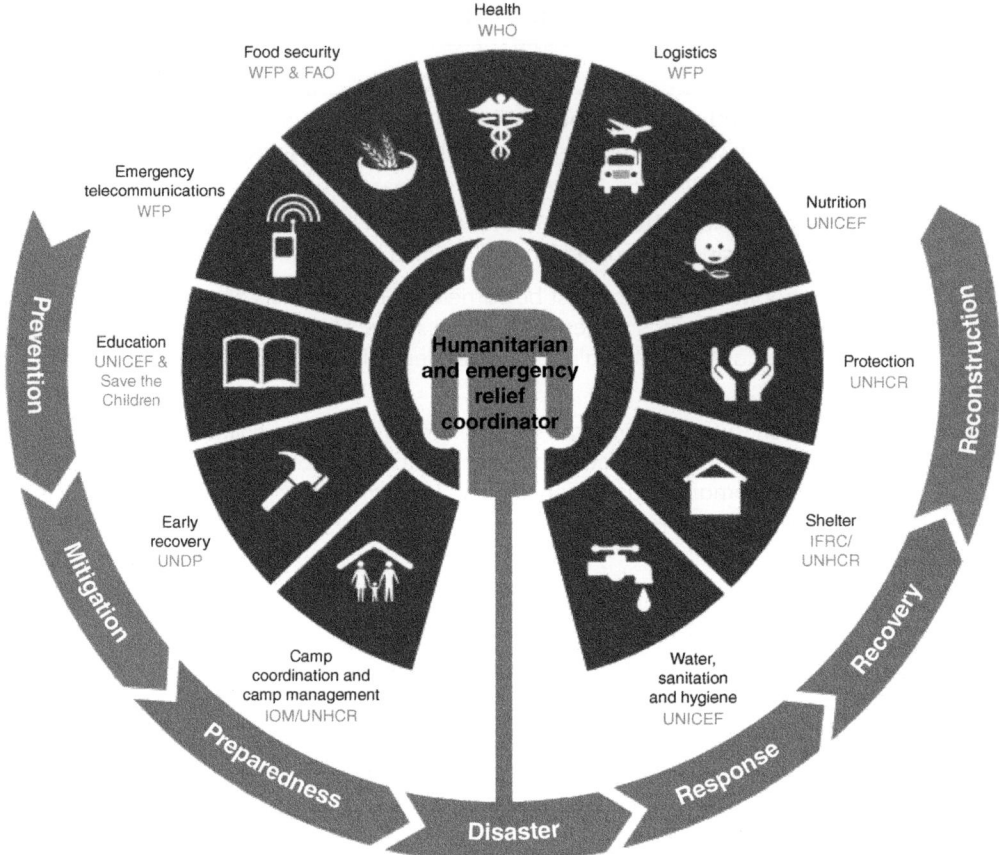

FIGURE 8.1   UN cluster system.

service providers (government, commercial, voluntary sector), iNGOs, and, possibly, military health services. A list of partners of the Global Health Cluster is available on the partners page of the WHO Health Cluster website.

THE INTERNATIONAL HUMANITARIAN HEALTH RESPONSE

There are a large number of national and iNGOs who coordinate and deliver health services during humanitarian emergencies using a combination of paid and voluntary personnel. Major organisations include the International Committee of the Red Cross, the International Federation of Red Cross and Red Crescent Societies, Doctors without Borders, Save the Children, Malteser International, Project Hope, Medical Teams International and World Vision. Individual crises spawn multiple additional NGOs and voluntary organisations as a platform for international and local community support. This can create a complex market for grant funds, provision of services, employment of local and international health professionals, and public engagement. It also creates challenges in the coordination of the health response between the UN Health

Cluster, iNGOs, local NGOs, and national, regional, and local health authorities. Each humanitarian crisis and complex emergency presents common and unique problems for the provision of health services to meet the needs of affected populations. Table 8.2 lists some of the health crises of the 21st century that have influenced the behaviour and learning across stakeholders in the humanitarian health sector.

A review by de Ville de Goyet of lessons from earthquakes and tsunamis in the first decade of the 20th century identified a series of endemic challenges in the timely

TABLE 8.2   Examples of humanitarian crises with significant health impacts in the 21st century.

Example	Dates	Characteristics
Afghanistan war	Protracted complex emergency since 1970s	The US led counterinsurgency campaign (2001–2021) resulted in significant changes to perspectives in civil–military relations
Iraq war	2003 onwards	US-led invasion in 2003 changed the balance of political power including a war against ISIS in 2013–2017. Healthcare was a significant political pawn
Bam, Iran earthquake	2003	Multi-national international response
Asia-Pacific tsunami	2004	Multi-national international response across many affected countries
Pakistan earthquake	2005	Multi-national international response with suggestions of disruption to local health economies.
Haiti earthquake	2010	Chaotic national and international response and persistent insecurity
Syrian civil war	2011 onwards	Civil war plus international interventions resulted in a major refugee crisis and evidence of attacks on healthcare
West Africa Ebola outbreak	2014–2016	Call for significant military contribution to international response. Recurrent outbreaks in DRC since 2018
Yemen civil war	2014 onwards	Multi-lateral civil war with significant destruction of health services
War in Ukraine	2014 onwards	Russian invasion in 2014 and escalation in 2022 that resulted in largest refugee crisis in Europe since Second World War
COVID-19 pandemic	2019–2023	Largest pandemic since influenza pandemic of 1918
Sudan	2023 onwards	Endemic political tension resulted in civil war and a humanitarian crisis
Israel–Hamas conflict	Enduring; upsurge of violence in 2023	Endemic political conflict with substantial escalation in violence since October 2023

management of the international response [6]. Foreign medical teams rarely arrive in time with suitable capabilities to provide immediate trauma care, though they can contribute to the secondary clinical management of survivors. Donations of medical equipment and supplies may not comply with established guidelines with much material having to be destroyed after arrival. The risk of epidemics may be overstated with community immunisation programmes distracting from the more important task of restoring safe water supplies and sanitation. Local medical volunteers may be usurped by international volunteers. A literature review by Arnaouti et al. in 2020 of observations from the international response to the earthquake in Haiti showed similar findings [7]. Although many lives were saved, there were challenges in coordination across national and international actors, some responders were insufficiently trained and experienced for their role, and local Haitian stakeholders were marginalised. A review of the local and international response to the Ebola outbreak in West Africa in 2014 also exposed some shortcomings in the global system for responding to health emergencies, coordination across international and local stakeholders, and the importance of community engagement [8]. There are similar analyses for the other humanitarian crises listed in Table 8.2.

There is a particular challenge for the relationship and coordination of the response in humanitarian crises and complex emergencies between civil and military actors. Armed forces, by their very nature, cannot be neutral nor operationally independent (as they are under the control of governments). However, they may have significant capabilities (command and control, logistics, medical services) that could be of significant assistance as part of an overall response. This has been highlighted in observations and studies from the wars in Iraq and Afghanistan and the responses to natural disasters such as the earthquake in Haiti and the Ebola outbreak of 2014. UN OCHA hosts a range of resources to guide civil–military coordination during humanitarian emergencies [9]. The WHO published a guidance document for civil–military coordination as part of health emergency preparedness in 2021 based on the Sendai Framework and observations from outbreaks of infectious diseases during the second decade of the 20th century [10].

Observations and lessons from the international humanitarian response have shown the importance of standards, guidelines, and normative agreements to ensure the best possible health outcomes for populations affected by humanitarian disasters, complex emergencies, and war. These should be adopted by local and international organisations at both a system level and also as a framework for the training and education of their personnel.

SPHERE HANDBOOK HEALTH SYSTEM STANDARDS

This book, and specifically this part of the book, is based on the structure of the health section of the Sphere Handbook.[3] The Sphere project is a multi-decade endeavour to improve the quality of humanitarian responses by promoting 'minimum standards' for each element of the four technical services to be provided as part of humanitarian response (water supply, sanitation and hygiene promotion; food security and nutrition; shelter and settlement; health). It builds upon the humanitarian principles and sets out the humanitarian charter as the ethical and legal foundations for the protection, behaviours, and standards of organisations and people working in the humanitarian sector. It emphasises three rights of all people affected by a disaster or conflict: the right to life with dignity; the right to receive humanitarian assistance; and the right of civilians and non-combatants to protection and security. The four protection principles build upon a human rights perspective and state the purpose of humanitarian action:

- to enhance the safety, dignity and rights of people, and avoid exposing them to harm;
- to ensure people's access to assistance according to need and without discrimination;
- to assist people to recover from the physical and psychological effects of threatened or actual violence, coercion or deliberate deprivation; and
- to help people claim their rights.

The Core Humanitarian Standard describes nine commitments for organisations and staff undertaking humanitarian activities to develop the quality and effectiveness of the services that they provide.

HEALTH SYSTEMS AND STANDARDS

The Health Chapter of the Sphere Handbook covers health systems and then the seven clinical dimensions of essential healthcare:

- communicable diseases;
- child health;
- sexual and reproductive health;
- injury and trauma care;
- mental health;
- non-communicable disease; and
- palliative care

This list provides the content of the remainder of this section of the book, though the order has been changed to reflect the timeline of the impact of war on health described in Chapter 3. The Sphere standards for health systems cover the five core aspects of a well-functioning health system:

- delivery of quality health services;
- a trained and motivated healthcare workforce;
- appropriate supply, management and use of medicines, diagnostics material and technology;
- appropriate financing of healthcare; and
- good health information and analysis.

This list mirrors the WHO building blocks for a health system described in Chapter 1. However, achieving the standards described in the Sphere Handbook is unlikely to occur during the immediate humanitarian response to a crisis. Rather, they set the direction of travel in the transition from emergency response to medium-term recovery and development as the health system recovers. The integration of concepts from emergency preparedness with concepts from health system capacity building is described in the implementation guide for health systems recovery in emergencies published by the WHO Regional Office for the Eastern Mediterranean [11].

In addition to subordinate standards for the seven clinical services in the Sphere Handbook, the WHO and other international reference bodies publish technical guidance for such services in humanitarian and emergency settings. An example is the suite of material published by WHO for international emergency medical teams (EMTs) that have been created to address the wide variation in competence and performance of EMTs that have arrived as part of the response to health emergencies in the past [12]. This material includes the 'Red Book' [13] that is used as a framework for verification and accreditation of international medical teams and the 'Blue Book' [14] with the full list of technical standards for each type of EMT. Relevant clinical guidance documents will be included in each of the subsequent chapters in this section of the book.

The development of standards and guidance should be based on research evidence of the effects of health interventions. Undertaking such research can be very challenging due to the risks to researchers and the difficulties of collecting data. The Humanitarian Health Evidence Review study team has published two systematic reviews to assess the evidence base for public health interventions in humanitarian crises [15, 16]. These show that there has been an increase in the number of publications evaluating the effectiveness of humanitarian health interventions, but there are gaps in coverage and methodology, and barriers in achieving equity across affected populations. The issues and challenges associated with conducting research in health during insecurity and war will be examined in Chapter 13. Please undertake Learning Activity 8.2 to examine the health system response in a contemporary complex emergency.

> **Learning Activity 8.2   Case Study – Health Systems Response to Humanitarian Crises – Syria**
>
> Building upon the literature search that you undertook for Learning Activity 3.2 about academic publications from the Syrian civil war, conduct a literature search on the challenges associated with the health systems response to meet the needs of populations affected by the Syrian civil war.
>
> You can compare your findings with the 'key points' summary at the end of the chapter.

ATTACKS ON HEALTHCARE

Unfortunately, healthcare personnel, transports, and facilities may be attacked and damaged during conflict. Chapter 6 summarised International Humanitarian Law (IHL) and emphasised the protections specifically afforded to health facilities, transports, and personnel. The second decade of the 21st century might be characterised by conflicts in which the protagonists clearly had no restraints to the manner by which they waged war. This particularly affected access to healthcare as at least one party seemed to explicitly attack healthcare facilities with the intention of undermining the will of the dependent population to resist their enemy. The war in Syria also saw the first use of chemical weapons by a state actor in the 21st century. The disruption of governance in northern Syria and north-western Iraq led to the creation of the so-called Islamic State of Iraq by the group known as ISIS. ISIS waged a war of terror including the mistreatment and murder of prisoners and the attempted genocide of the Yazidi population. The counter-ISIS operations undertaken by the Iraqi government, supported by a US-led international coalition, involved some very difficult battles in urban areas, most particularly Mosul. The arrangements for medical care for the combat forces, the civilian population, and captured ISIS prisoners generated some complex debates over responsibilities for the provision of healthcare under IHL to each of these groups. It could be argued that the international consensus concerning the purposes of the Geneva Conventions and IHL is under serious strain. Therefore, the rights of protection and the rights of humanitarian access for non-combatants are not being respected. This is most evident by the direct targeting and destruction of healthcare facilities during the conflict, though there are also secondary methods to attack healthcare, for example cyberattacks on health information services or subjecting healthcare professionals to intimidation or murder.

These threats to healthcare systems question the effectiveness of the Red Cross or other Geneva emblems as a protective symbol. It is possible that healthcare leaders in conflict environments will need to consider passive and active measures to protect healthcare facilities. Passive measures might include ballistic protection (sandbags and concrete barriers), underground bunkers, and minimalising electronic transmission (such as banning mobile phones). Active measures might include the specific protection of medical facilities by security forces and the use of weapons to protect against missile and drone attacks. This poses the question of whether the concept of humanitarian space remains valid, or indeed whether there is a difference between military and civilian healthcare during conflict amongst the people. Two United Nations resolutions have strongly condemned attacks and threats against healthcare and civilians, and have called upon armed actors to comply with IHL [17]. The WHO established an initiative on stopping attacks on healthcare [18]. It defines an attack on healthcare as any act of verbal or physical violence or obstruction or threat of violence that interferes with the availability, access and delivery of curative and/or preventive health services during emergencies. Types of attacks vary across contexts and can range from violence with heavy weapons to psychosocial threats and intimidation. The WHO published practical guidance for the prevention and protection against attacks on healthcare in 2023 [19]. In parallel, the International Committee of the Red Cross (ICRC) established the Healthcare in Danger project and has also published many advocacy and guidance documents on the application of IHL to ensure access to healthcare and protect health services during conflict [20].

LOOKING FORWARD

This chapter has outlined how health systems respond to insecurity or crises both at a local or national level, and also as part of an international system. The role of the UN in humanitarian crises has been described. The Sphere Handbook has been summarised to set the context for the subsequent chapters in this section. Key sources of guidance for the role of health systems in response to the health impact amongst populations affected by humanitarian emergencies have been provided. The next chapter will look at how health systems are organised to care for trauma patients from the point of injury to rehabilitation and recovery.

SOURCES AND RESOURCES

Suggested Internet search strings are as follows: 'health systems war'; 'health systems humanitarian'; 'health systems recovery'; 'health systems resilience'; and 'health systems emergency response'.

UN OCHA, available at https://www.unocha.org/. This is a website for the United Nations Office for the Coordination of Humanitarian Affairs (OCHA).

UNICEF Health in Emergencies, available at https://www.unicef.org/health/emergencies

WHO websites:

Emergency Medical Teams, available at https://www.who.int/emergencies/partners/emergency-medical-teams

Health Emergencies, available at https://www.who.int/our-work/health-emergencies

Global Health Emergencies, available at https://www.who.int/emergencies/overview

Health Cluster, available at https://healthcluster.who.int/

Alliance for Health Policy and Systems Research, available at https://ahpsr.who.int/

Pan American Health Organisation – Health Emergency and Disaster Preparedness, available at https://www.paho.org/en/topics/health-emergency-and-disaster-preparedness

International Federation of Red Cross and Red Crescent Societies, available at Emergency Health. https://www.ifrc.org/our-work/health-and-care/emergency-health

Rapid Health Assessment of Refugee or Displaced Populations (3rd edition). 2006. Medecins Sans Frontiers. Available at http://refbooks.msf.org/msf_docs/en/rapid_health/rapid_health_en.pdf

ERLA, available at https://www.elrha.org/. A global research network that finds solutions to complex humanitarian problems through research and innovation.

Centre for Humanitarian Health, available at https://hopkinshumanitarianhealth.org/. A global research and education network to pursue knowledge and disseminate learning to save lives and reduce suffering in humanitarian emergencies.

Geneva Centre of Humanitarian Studies, available at https://humanitarianstudies.ch/. The Geneva Centre of Humanitarian Studies is a platform for teaching, research, and dialogue in the field of humanitarian action.

Harvard Humanitarian Initiative, available at https://hhi.harvard.edu/home. This is a university-wide academic and research centre in humanitarian crisis and leadership.

ReBUILD, available at https://www.rebuildconsortium.com/. ReBUILD for Resilience examines health system resilience in fragile settings experiencing violence, conflict, pandemics and other shocks.

MEDBOX, available at https://www.medbox.org/. MEDBOX is an online library of guidelines, textbooks and practical documents for healthcare in a humanitarian setting.

Learning Activity 8.2 Case Study – Health Systems Response to Humanitarian Crises – Syria – Key Point Summary

Hopefully, you will have made a table using the WHO building block structure, from Chapter 1 that looks something like the one below.

Topic	Citations	Key points
Leadership/governance		
Service delivery		
Health workforce		
Information		
Medical products, vaccines, technologies		
Financing		
Health outcomes		

You might also have found some papers that reported health outcomes as a consequence of the war and added an additional row. Rather than show a worked version in this chapter which will be out of date when you undertake this Learning Activity for yourself, it is suggested that you compare your findings with the paper by Haar et al. [21] which is a qualitative study of interviews with 40 healthcare workers with direct experience of the impacts of the war in Northern Syria.

APPENDIX A   Figure 8.2

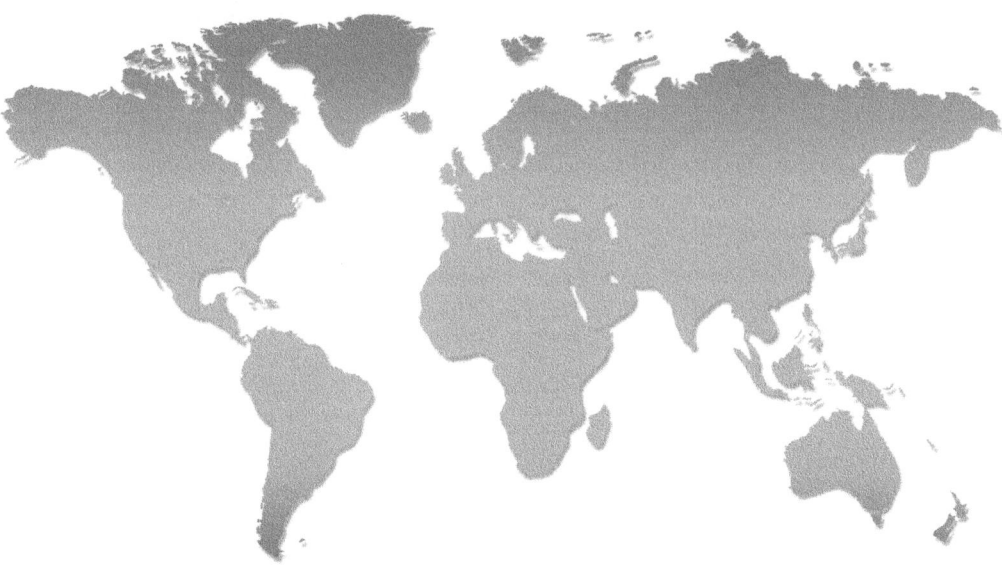

FIGURE 8.2   World map.

NOTES

1. The Sendai Framework is available at `https://www.undrr.org/implementing-sendai-framework`.
2. Bangkok Principles for the implementation of the health aspects of the Sendai Framework for Disaster Risk Reduction 2015–2030. Available at `https://www.undrr.org/media/17231/download?startDownload=20240613`; a series of WHO factsheets on difference health domains of emergency and disaster risk management (EDRM) are available at `https://www.who.int/publications/m/item/health-emergency-and-disaster-risk-management-(edrm)-fact-sheets`.
3. Sphere Handbook. Available at: `https://handbook.spherestandards.org/en/sphere/`.

REFERENCES

1. WHO (2019). *Health Emergency and Disaster Risk Management Framework.* Geneva: World Health Organization. Licence: CC BY-NC-SA 3.0 IGO. `https://iris.who.int/bitstream/handle/10665/326106/9789241516181-eng.pdf?sequence=1` (accessed 29 March 2025).
2. WHO (2023). *Strengthening Health Emergency Prevention, Preparedness, Response and Resilience.* Geneva: World Health Organization. `https://cdn.who.int/media/docs/default-source/emergency-preparedness/who_hepr_wha2023-21051248b.pdf` (accessed 29 March 2025).

3. UN (1991). Strengthening the Coordination of Humanitarian Emergency Assistance of the United Nations. UN General Assembly Resolution 46/182. New York: United Nations. https://undocs.org/Home/Mobile?FinalSymbol=A%2FRES%2F46%2F182&Language=E&DeviceType=Desktop&LangRequested=False (accessed 29 March 2025).

4. UN OCHA (2022). *What are Humanitarian Principles? OCHA on Message.* New York: UN OCHA. https://www.unocha.org/publications/report/world/ocha-message-humanitarian-principles (accessed 29 March 2025).

5. WHO (2021). *Health Cluster Guide: A Practical Handbook.* Geneva: World Health Organisation. https://library.alnap.org/help-library/health-cluster-guide-a-practical-handbook. The WHO Health Cluster website is at: https://healthcluster.who.int/ (accessed 29 March 2025).

6. de Goyet, C.V. (2007). Health lessons learned from the recent earthquakes and Tsunami in Asia. *Prehospital and Disaster Medicine* 22 (1): 15–21. https://doi.org/10.1017/s1049023x00004283.

7. Arnaouti, M.K., Cahill, G., Baird, M.D. et al. (2022). Medical disaster response: a critical analysis of the 2010 Haiti earthquake. *Frontiers in Public Health* 10: 995595. https://doi.org/10.3389/fpubh.2022.995595.

8. Coltart, C.E., Lindsey, B., Ghinai, I. et al. (2017). The Ebola outbreak, 2013–2016: old lessons for new epidemics. *Philosophical Transactions of the Royal Society B: Biological Sciences* 372 (1721): 20160297. http://dx.doi.org/10.1098/rstb.2016.0297.

9. Civil-Military Coordination. UN OCHA. https://www.unocha.org/civil-military-coordination (accessed 2 April 2025).

10. WHO (2021). *National Civil–Military Health Collaboration Framework for Strengthening Health Emergency Preparedness: WHO Guidance Document.* Geneva: World Health Organization. https://iris.who.int/bitstream/handle/10665/343571/9789240030343-eng.pdf?sequence=1 (accessed 2 April 2025).

11. WHO (2020). *Implementation Guide for Health Systems Recovery in Emergencies: Transforming Challenges into Opportunities.* Cairo: WHO Regional Office for the Eastern Mediterranean. https://applications.emro.who.int/docs/9789290223351-eng.pdf?ua=1 (accessed 2 April 2025).

12. WHO. *Emergency Medical Teams.* WHO Website. https://www.who.int/emergencies/partners/emergency-medical-teams (accessed 2 April 2025).

13. WHO (2021). *A Guidance Document for Medical Teams Responding to Health Emergencies in Armed Conflicts and Other Insecure Environments.* Geneva: World Health Organization. https://www.who.int/publications/i/item/9789240029354 (accessed 2 April 2025).

14. WHO (2021). *Classification and Minimum Standards for Emergency Medical Teams.* Geneva: World Health Organization. https://www.who.int/publications/i/item/9789240029330 (accessed 2 April 2025).

15. Blanchet, K., Sistenich, V., Ramesh, A., et al. (2013). *An Evidence Review of Research on Health Interventions in Humanitarian Crises.* Cardiff, UK: Enhancing Learning

and Research for Humanitarian Assistance (ELRHA). https://www.elrha.org/wp-content/uploads/2015/01/Evidence-Review-22.10.15.pdf (accessed 2 April 2025).

16. Doocy, S., Lyles, E., Tappis, H. et al. (2023). Effectiveness of humanitarian health interventions: a systematic review of literature published between 2013 and 2021. *BMJ Open* 13 (7): e068267. https://doi.org/10.1136/bmjopen-2022-068267.

17. (a) UNSCR S/RES/2286 (2016). https://undocs.org/S/RES/2286(2016); (b) UNSC S/RES/2730 (2024). https://undocs.org/S/RES/2730(2024).

18. WHO. *Initiative Stopping Attacks on Healthcare.* https://www.who.int/activities/stopping-attacks-on-health-care (accessed 2 April 2025).

19. WHO (2023). *Prevention and Protection Against Attacks on Health Care: Good Practices.* Geneva: World Health Organization. https://www.who.int/publications/i/item/9789240019461 (accessed 2 April 2025).

20. ICRC. *Healthcare in Danger.* Geneva: ICRC. https://healthcareindanger.org/ (accessed 2 April 2025).

21. Haar, R., Rayes, D., Tappis, H. et al. (2024). The cascading impacts of attacks on health in Syria: a qualitative study of health system and community impacts. *PLOS Global Public Health* 4 (6): e0002967. https://doi.org/10.1371/journal.pgph.0002967.

CHAPTER 9

War and Physical Trauma

Eddie Chaloner and Martin Bricknell

Centre for Conflict and Health Security, King's College London, London, UK

Abstract

The aim of this chapter is to describe the provision of clinical services to care for physical trauma patients in war. Chapter 3 described the impact of war on health, and Chapter 5 covered how weapons are designed to kill and maim. This chapter shows how health services can be organised to mitigate these effects on physical trauma. Trauma services will be presented as a 'chain of care' from the point of injury to rehabilitation and recovery. Each element will be summarised with an emphasis on the organisation of the whole system. It will link to the previous chapter about health systems' response to crisis and also emphasise that trauma is not the only source of medical emergencies, even during conflict. It will close by highlighting some sources of detailed technical information to help healthcare practitioners be prepared for war casualties. It should be noted that psychological trauma will be considered in Chapter 13.

Keywords: chain of care, triage, damage control, war surgery, rehabilitation

Handbook of Global Health, Security, and War, First Edition. Edited by Martin Bricknell and Richard Sullivan.
© 2025 John Wiley & Sons Ltd. Published 2025 by John Wiley & Sons Ltd.

KEY LEARNING OUTCOMES

By studying this chapter, the reader will be able to:

- Describe the organisation of trauma care during the war as a 'chain of care'
- Summarise the particular skills required of healthcare professionals at each stage of the 'chain of care'
- Explain the importance of rehabilitation and recovery services for the restoration of maximum health for trauma patients

---

INTRODUCTION

Chapter 3 described the major primary impacts of conflict on health as death and injuries from weapons. Chapter 5 explained that the agents that affect human health during the war can be classified using the mnemonic CBRNE3T, **c**hemical, **b**iological, **r**adiological, **n**uclear (CBRN), **e**xplosive, **e**ndemic, **e**nvironmental, and non-battle **t**rauma. The effects of weapons on the human body depend on the type of weapon and the part of the body that has been attacked. This chapter will consider how services to care for physical trauma can mitigate some of the explosive effects on the human body.

This chapter is based upon Section 2.4 Injury and Trauma Care of the Health Chapter in the Sphere Handbook at pages 335–339. The demand for physical trauma services in time of war is highly likely to exceed the routine capacity of local health systems in terms of clinical expertise, volume of medical facilities, and medical logistics. Therefore, the health system will need to establish triage (the prioritisation of casualties according to clinical need) and mass casualty management across the whole system providing emergency, operative, nursing, and rehabilitative care. Much depends on the capacity and training of the health system in trauma management before the conflict broke out. Systems accustomed to managing war or non-war-related trauma on a regular basis generally adapt faster to the outbreak of acute conflict. Medical logistics and supply chain management have a major influence on the ability of a system to manage a surge in demand. In peacetime, healthcare systems do not carry large stocks of the type of consumables needed to deal with substantial volumes of severely injured patients and supplies can rapidly be exhausted. The key actions for injury and physical trauma care during a humanitarian emergency are to[1]:

- Provide care for trauma at all levels for all patients
- Ensure that healthcare workers have the skills and knowledge to address injuries
- Establish or strengthen standardised protocols for triage and injury and trauma care
- Provide tetanus prophylaxis to anyone at risk of injury, to injured people with open wounds, and to those involved in rescue operations
- Ensure minimum safety and governance standards for all facilities providing trauma and injury care, including field hospitals

- Ensure timely access to rehabilitation services, priority assistive devices, and mobility aids for injured patients
- Establish or strengthen the health information systems to include injury and trauma data

Trauma systems comprise a chain of facilities and expertise to handle emergencies using a standardised approach to the management of patients with life and limb-threatening injuries. Whilst the care of physical trauma is likely to be at the centre of the health response during conflict, other health emergencies, such as the COVID-19 pandemic, emphasised the importance of a holistic approach to clinical emergencies. The World Health Organization (WHO) Emergency, Trauma and Acute Care programme champions these services as an essential element of Universal Health Coverage. It provides a range of resources to support the development of emergency health systems including detailed clinical guidance for each element [1]. This chapter will cite multiple resources from this programme as examples of guidelines or reference documents for trauma care. A scoping literature review by Werner et al. identified gaps in prehospital care delivery, transport, and initial reception and management in emergency departments (EDs) of hospitals in emergency care systems in fragile and conflict-affected settings [2]. Key barriers to development included lingering social distrust amongst conflict-affected communities, scarcity of formal training in emergency care, poor infrastructure, and lack of resources and supplies.

War, as an epidemic of injuries, often leads to advances in trauma care by military health services that are translated into civilian practice. Historical innovations include the development of the ambulance, first aid training, X-rays, blood transfusion, adoption of penicillin as an antibiotic, and reconstructive surgical techniques in orthopaedics and plastic surgery. In 'Western' health systems, lessons from military medicine resulting from caring for casualties during the wars in Iraq and Afghanistan have been translated into civilian practice within home nations and many of these are transferable to global practice [3].

Chapter 6 discussed attacks on healthcare and the threats faced by healthcare professionals, ambulances, and facilities during conflict. Unfortunately, this means that safety and security is a critical principle in the organisation of trauma services. Personnel involved in the provision and leadership of trauma services must be competent to identify hazards, mitigate risks to personal safety, and ultimately decide not to provide services if the risks to healthcare personnel are too great. Many international non-government organisations (NGOs) insist that all their personnel undertake formal hazardous environment training before deploying as part of a humanitarian response. Local healthcare workers should also receive equivalent training. They may need to be issued with helmets and body armour alongside their insignia that identifies them as members of a humanitarian organisation, although in certain circumstances this can also identify them as a target.

'CHAINS OF CARE'

Trauma services can be considered as a 'chain of care' through which a trauma patient passes with increasingly sophisticated levels of clinical care alongside transport between each level of medical facility. Please complete Learning Activity 9.1 to examine the elements of a 'chain of care'.

Learning Activity 9.1   Chains of Care

Review the images that summarise a trauma system in each of the following documents. Describe the similarities and differences between the images.

WHO (2018). *WHO Emergency Care System Framework.* Available at: https://www.who.int/publications/i/item/who-emergency-care-system-framework.

Figure 1 in Garber, K., Kushner, A.L., Wren, S.M. et al. (2020). Applying trauma systems concepts to humanitarian battlefield care: a qualitative analysis of the Mosul trauma pathway. *Conflict and Health* 14: 5. Available at: https://doi.org/10.1186/s13031-019-0249-2.

Page 6 of Operational Response for Gaza (2019). Ongoing health response & 96-hour Contingency Planning. Gerald Rockenschaub, Head of West Bank & Gaza. https://www.emro.who.int/images/stories/palestine/documents/final_health_cluster_-_gaza_ongoing_needs__96_hr_contingency_plan_11mar19.pdf.

Halimah, S. *WHO Health Cluster Coordinator.* https://reliefweb.int/sites/reliefweb.int/files/resources/final_health_cluster_-_gaza_ongoing_needs_96_hr_contingency_plan_11mar19.pdf.

Figure 3 in Bricknell, M. (2014). For debate: the operational patient care pathway. *BMJ Military Health* 160: 64–69. https://militaryhealth.bmj.com/content/160/1/64.

Suggested answers are at the end of the chapter.

This learning activity has shown that clinical services for the treatment of physical trauma comprise a 'pre-hospital' phase, a 'hospital phase', and a 'rehabilitation and recovery phase'. These phases are joined together by an ambulance system and a 'command and control' system. Many of the concepts within a 'chain of care' originate from lessons learned in military health services. This chapter will now consider each of these phases and their subordinate elements.

PRE-HOSPITAL CARE

This section will consider the components of a pre-hospital care system including first aid, ambulance (or evacuation), resuscitation or stabilisation points, and a command-and-control system. Each will be considered in turn.

First Aid

First aid is the start of the 'chain of care'. This is usually provided by a bystander and includes the 'call for help'. Pre-hospital first aid skills are often taught as: scene safety, calling for help, stopping massive bleeding, protection of the airway, support to breathing, and compressing external bleeding. Two mnemonics are in widespread use to help first aiders remember their priorities for assessment and treatment: **MARCH**, **m**assive bleeding, **a**irway, **r**espiration, **c**irculation, **h**eat (prevent and treat hot and cold injuries); or **< C > ABC**, **<c**atastrophic bleeding>, **a**irway, **b**reathing, and circulation. Armed forces often include first aid training as a mandatory, generic skill for all military personnel. An example is the US military Tactical Combat Casualty Care (TCCC) framework which comprises skills for the three phases of TCCC: **Care Under Fire, Tactical Field Care, Tactical Evacuation** (TACEVAC).[2] Repeated training and practice is particularly important because prior practice on an individual and group level serves to embed drills and standardised protocols which may otherwise be forgotten in the stress of conflict. Organisations such as the International Federation of Red Cross and Red Crescent Societies (IFRC) and the International Committee of the Red Cross (ICRC) publish first-aid handbooks and run training courses in first aid for the public and volunteers [4].[3,4]

Ambulance

A key role in first aid is calling for help and planning for the patient to travel to a higher level of care. Ambulances will often be crewed with a driver and a separate paramedic or other defined clinical provider. However, the coverage and competence of ambulance services vary considerably across the globe with some countries, especially fragile and conflict-affected states, having very limited public ambulance services. Patients may have to travel long distances at their own initiative in order to access healthcare, using taxis, pick-up trucks, or other improvised modes of transport without any additional care beyond bystander first aid.

Resuscitation and Stabilisation

In areas of high demand and long evacuation times, fixed or mobile medical teams may deploy to provide initial resuscitation and stabilisation prior to further evacuation of the patient to hospital-level care (for X-rays, blood transfusion, surgery, etc.). This tier might be the same as the 'primary care' tier of care described in Chapter 1, the health post or community clinic. The personnel that staff these facilities need to be able to manage health emergencies as well as providing community-based public health, preventive medicine services, and ambulatory primary care services. The education of these health professionals usually extends the previous mnemonics to cover a *primary* survey – **a**irway, **b**reathing, **c**irculation, **d**isability, and **e**xposure (**ABCDE**) – and a *secondary* survey to detect other clinically important injuries. Ideally, these skills would match those of the health professionals employed in the ED of the hospital, but in the initial phases of war in an 'unprimed' healthcare system facing large numbers of civilian casualties, this standard is rarely met in practice. In times of great and prolonged stress to a health system, some practitioners may be required to act above their normal level of training and outside their area of normal clinical expertise. Further, experienced practitioners accustomed to working in peacetime structures may need to rapidly adapt to changed physical circumstances and resource constraints. One example of the need for new skill acquisition is the importance of limb tourniquets in wartime to reduce bleeding during prolonged evacuation. Tourniquet devices are rarely needed in peacetime trauma but can be a lifesaver in wartime. However, they also can be hazardous if used incorrectly and not monitored.

Command and Control

Some of the examples of 'chains of care' discussed in Learning Activity 8.1 explicitly included a command-and-control system that organises ambulance despatch and notification of hospitals. In developed countries, these may involve sophisticated 'tactical control centres' that coordinate the response to calls from the public by assigning a spectrum of different ambulance capabilities, possibly including helicopter-borne, doctor-led emergency teams. There are a number of training systems which cover the skills for this element of the pre-hospital system, including the UK Major Incident Medical Management and Support (MIMMS).[5] Training for MIMMS uses a mnemonic **CSCATTT** (**C**ommand and **C**ontrol, **S**afety, **C**ommunications, **A**ssessment, **T**riage, **T**reatment, **T**ransport) to cover all of the organisational functions that need to occur in the pre-hospital phase of trauma care. This includes the specific function of Triage.

Triage

Triage, using the French word meaning 'to sort', covers the action of sorting and prioritising patients based on an estimation of the clinical urgency for initial treatment and subsequent evacuation or further treatment. It can be performed at any point in the care of patients, including in both pre-hospital ambulance services and hospitals, where patients have to be 'sequenced' for their access to the next level of clinical service. The WHO-sponsored Interagency Integrated Triage Tool is an example of an agreed categorisation system for triage across many humanitarian agencies [5]. Triage in practice also relates to the capacity of the system to meet demand. In times when surge capacity is exceeded, triage thresholds will change, often significantly, and this may eventually be reflected in poorer clinical outcomes compared to before the emergency.

HOSPITAL CARE

Hospital care requires functioning hospitals that are orientated to receiving and treating emergency patients. Hospitals are complex 'socio-technical' organisations that require sophisticated organisational and managerial structures that coordinate the six building blocks of a health system (from Chapter 1) into an effective clinical organisation. Whilst a relatively old publication, the ICRC guide for running a hospital for war-wounded remains a valid summary of the issues and challenges that need to be addressed by the hospital leadership team [6]. This includes all of the human resource and logistic elements of hospital management alongside the procedures to adjust clinical services to respond to a surge in physical trauma cases. This section will cover the three clinical areas of a hospital that will be most involved in responding to physical trauma cases: the ED, the operating department, and the 'nursing department' including the critical care area.

Emergency Department

Learning Activity 9.1 showed that a health system should be designed to manage all types of health emergencies, not just trauma. It is important to appreciate that civilian healthcare requirements continue during wartime with the same incidence – the demands of war are in addition to normal requirements. Non-trauma emergencies include emergencies such as a heart attack, meningitis, septic shock, stroke, diabetic coma, and obstetric emergencies. During conflict, clinical services for non-trauma emergencies must not be usurped by trauma care insofar as is possible and practical. In ideal circumstances, all hospitals should have a clearly demarcated ED as the location for reception (or 'booking-in'), triage, and assignment of clinical area for all emergency patients. T1 (the most severe cases) would be assigned to the resuscitation area where staff, equipment, medications, and processes are organised to allow emergency interventions to be delivered efficiently. T2 patients may be assigned to a lower care area in the ED or rapidly processed for admission to another clinical area, such as a pre-designated nursing ward. T3 patients can be treated after the surge of patients has been cleared. They might be held outside the ED or redirected to community primary care services.

The initial phase of resuscitation should follow standardised procedures similar to the structure used for first aid. The WHO trauma resuscitation algorithm is an example of a widely used format that uses the ABCDE approach [7]. It can be taught to all members of the resuscitation team so that everyone understands the common approach and can support each other in the care of the most severe patients. Treatment plans for specific clinical emergencies can be standardised into checklists which can be used as an aide-memoire, similar to a pilots' checklist for flying. Examples are the WHO Trauma Care Checklist [8] and the WHO Medical Emergencies Checklist [9].

Operating Department

The operating department covers the clinical functions of surgery, anaesthesia, and post-operative recovery. Military medicine has been driven by the specialist operative skills needed to manage war wounds. Many books have been written on the topic of War Surgery. These cover the general management of the war injured and the specific surgical techniques required to repair war wounds. The two volume, ICRC War Surgery: Working with Limited Resources in Armed Conflict and Other Situations of Violence, is an authoritative reference manual on all aspects of War Surgery (cited in the Sources and Resources section of this chapter). If the ED has been able to address threats to the patient's airway and breathing and been able to stem external bleeding, the majority of early deaths from war wounds in hospital are attributed to non-compressible bleeding in the skull, chest, abdomen, and pelvis which can only be stopped by a surgical procedure. War injuries can be very complex, involving multiple limbs and body cavities. Often it is not possible to undertake all the surgical interventions needed by a patient in one visit to the operating theatre as it may also be too time-consuming if other patients are waiting for surgery. The concepts of **damage control resuscitation (DCR) and damage control surgery (DCS)** address the challenges of dealing with complex multiple injuries in a stepwise fashion in order of priority [10].

DCR has been defined as a systematic approach to dealing with major trauma combining the catastrophic bleeding, airway, breathing, and circulation paradigm with a series of clinical techniques from immediate lifesaving measures up to surgical interventions in order to minimise blood loss, maximise tissue oxygenation, and deliver the patient to the operating theatre in the best possible physiological state. This extends resuscitation concepts across the 'chain of care' from the point of injury into the operating and critical care departments. It reinforces the need for integrated approaches toward resuscitation between the clinical specialities of emergency medicine, anaesthesia, and critical care.

DCS works on the principle of doing the minimal intervention required to stabilise the patient at each stage of the surgical process. DCS concepts recognise that after severe bleeding has been stopped and major bowel injuries have been externalised, most patients can be physiologically resuscitated and evacuated to a location for definitive correction of anatomical injury. Simply put, it is neither necessary nor desirable to correct all the damage immediately. Adopting a staged approach based on prioritisation generally achieves better outcomes. A well-functioning DCS system reduces the logistic load on forward units but relies on astute surgical and anaesthetic decision-making combined with collaborative teamwork with critical care colleagues. A patient who has undergone DCS will require post-operative critical care and is highly likely to require at least one subsequent operation within a very short period.

The history of War Surgery has been dominated by the risk of wound infection, especially the extensive contamination that occurs as a result of **temporary cavitation** caused by high-velocity fragments (link to the discussion on bullets in Chapter 5). This means that most wounds caused directly by high-energy transfer missiles or fragments need to undergo **primary surgery** to be thoroughly cleaned, **debrided** (removal of dead tissue), and left open for drainage. The surgeon should then review the wound around 4–7 days later and, if the wound is healthy, the wound can be closed. This technique is called **delayed primary closure (DPC)**. Even with DPC, war wounds can lead to deep tissue infection that may be extremely difficult to treat in spite of modern antibiotics especially if it involves bone. Repeated surgical procedures may be required. The prevalence of wound infections amongst the war wounded can lead to contamination of hospitals and the emergence of bacteria and fungi that are resistant to multiple antimicrobials. Antimicrobial resistance (AMR) was discussed in Chapter 5 on Global Health Security.

Nursing Department

This department covers both the critical care (or intensive care) area and the general nursing wards. Outcomes of care for war wounded are substantially affected by the quality of nursing care. Critical care nursing (including respiratory ventilation) is a highly sophisticated, technically demanding clinical role that is the province of specialist staff within developed health systems. In many conflict settings, there is neither the equipment, medical supplies, nor competence amongst nursing staff to provide this level of intensive medical and nursing care. This may result in a decision to provide palliative and supportive care for the most severely injured patients rather than a curative approach. Such decisions are very challenging and emotionally draining for doctors and nurses accustomed to working only in peacetime conditions.

Basic nursing care including dressing changes, pain management, care of pressure areas, and feeding/washing of patients all have a substantial impact on eventual outcomes. Trained and committed nurses are an essential part of successful surgery. The recovery and rehabilitation process starts in the post-operative ward. Prevention of post-operative infection, restoration of physical function, and emotional/psychological support for patients are the responsibility of conscientious nurses doing routine nursing care on a post-operative ward to a high standard.

REHABILITATION AND RECOVERY

The provision of clinical services for the rehabilitation and recovery of the war injured are often 'Cinderella' services that do not receive the same attention and funding as emergency hospital-based clinical services. Reconstructive surgery is vital for reintegrating wounded patients back into civilian society. Initial surgery, especially in relation to amputation, is frequently incomplete during the initial crisis. Stumps may need revision to permit the functional use of prostheses. Without a functioning prosthesis, a war-wounded amputee may be able to re-enter the workforce. Large numbers of amputees can become a major economic burden on post-conflict societies with disenchanted war wounded. Complex facial and ophthalmic reconstruction are also important to restore dignity after these injuries. Restoration of an injured person back to a useful and productive role in society relies on these post-emergency health and social services. Rehabilitation can be considered as a clinical function comprising physiotherapy, prosthetic services (artificial limbs and other aids), occupational therapy, and mental health. Recovery can be considered as the process of restoring physical, psychological, and social health to enable the maximum level of return to function within the patients' community setting including work, education, and domestic life. Many clinical and social lessons for supporting the rehabilitation and recovery of the war injured have been learned after wars, including the experience of NATO nations in caring for veterans from the war in Afghanistan. The WHO has recognised the importance of including rehabilitation within health emergency preparedness, readiness, response, and resilience[6] and has a discrete programme of work for this topic [11]. The field handbook, Early Rehabilitation in Conflicts and Disasters, published by the NGO Humanity and Inclusion is a good reference point for the issues to be considered in planning and delivering rehabilitation services [12].

GOVERNANCE AND DATA

In addition to the command-and-control function described earlier, trauma systems require active governance based on measures of clinical outcomes for patients. The advances in military medicine and the improvement in survival rates of the NATO military wounded were founded upon the creation of 'trauma registries' with standardised clinical data recorded on all casualties throughout their treatment within the chain of care. Recording accurate data informs better decision-making which ultimately translates into better clinical outcomes. Building upon this experience, many civilian trauma systems have created their own managed networks supported by clinical registries. An example is the US Joint Theatre Trauma Registry (JTTR). Reflecting these initiatives, the WHO has created the WHO Clinical Registry as a platform for systematically collecting, aggregating, and analysing case-based emergency care records using a standard clinical case record [13, 14]. Learning Activity 9.2 provides more information on the use of trauma registries to support quality improvement within trauma services.

Learning Activity 9.2   Case Study – Trauma Registries

This chapter has argued that clinical services for trauma care should be considered as whole system. The performance of the system should be measured using standardised data. Please read the following three academic articles and consider the opportunities and barriers associated with implementing an integrated trauma system.

Rosenkrantz, L., Schuurman, N., Arenas, C. et al. (2020). Maximizing the potential of trauma registries in low-income and middle-income countries. *Trauma Surgery & Acute Care Open* 5(1):e000469. https://doi.org/10.1136/tsaco-2020-000469.

Sawe, H.R., Reynolds, T.A., Weber, E.J. et al. (2020). Trauma care and capture rate of variables of World Health Organization data set for injury at regional hospitals in Tanzania: first steps to a national trauma registry. *BMC Emergency* 20:29 https://doi.org/10.1186/s12873-020-00325-y.

Spott, M.A., Kurkowski, C.R and Stockinger, Z. (2018). The joint trauma system: history in the making. *Military Medicine* 183(2):4–7. https://doi.org/10.1093/milmed/usy166.

Suggested answers are at the end of the chapter.

LOOKING FORWARD

This chapter has provided an overview to the design and clinical capabilities required as part of the health system response to physical trauma. It has shown how a 'chain of care' can be used to illustrate the concept and structure of the whole system from the point of injury to recovery. The next chapter will consider communicable diseases both as epidemic risk associated with conflict and as a discrete threat to security.

SOURCES AND RESOURCES

(some of these are the same as Chapter 5 because many manuals on trauma care also include information on mechanisms of injury)

Suggested Internet search terms are as follows: 'trauma systems', 'war surgery', 'damage control resuscitation', and 'damage control surgery'.

Suggested websites and online sources for further information:

Emergency care systems for universal health coverage: ensuring timely care for the acutely ill and injured. (2019) Resolution WHA72.16 Seventy-second World Health Assembly. https://www.who.int/publications/i/item/emergency-care-systems-for-universal-health-coverage-ensuring-timely-care-for-the-acutely-ill-and-injured

World Health Organization. Emergency Care at https://www.who.int/health-topics/emergency-care#tab=tab_1. These web pages provide access to information on the WHO's Emergency, Trauma and Acute Care programme. This programme is dedicated to strengthening the emergency care systems that serve as the first point of contact with the health system for so much of the world, and to supporting the development of quality, timely emergency care accessible to all.

Mock, C., Lormand, J.D., Goosen, J. et al. (2004). *WHO Guidelines for Essential Trauma Care*. Geneva: World Health Organization. `https://www.who.int/publications/i/item/guidelines-for-essential-trauma-care`.

Guidelines for War Surgery – Working With Limited Resources In Armed Conflict And Other Situations Of Violence Volume 1. (2020) ICRC, Geneva. Available at `https://shop.icrc.org/war-surgery-working-with-limited-resources-in-armed-conflict-and-other-situations-of-violence-volume-1-pdf-en.html`

War Surgery – Working With Limited Resources in Armed Conflict and Other Situations Of Violence Volume 2. (2020) ICRC, Geneva. Available at `https://shop.icrc.org/war-surgery-working-with-limited-resources-in-armed-conflict-and-other-situations-of-violence-volume-2-print-en.html`

Emergency War Surgery 5th Edition. (2018) Ed Cubano MA. Borden Institute, Fort Sam Houston, Texas. Available at `https://medcoe.army.mil/borden-tb-ews`

Blast Trauma Care: Course Manual (2020) ICRC, Geneva. Available at `https://www.icrc.org/en/publication/4500-blast-trauma-care-course-manual`

Joint Trauma System. The Department of Defense Centre for Excellence for Trauma. Available at: `https://jts.health.mil/`. The mission of the Joint Trauma System (JTS) is to improve trauma readiness and outcomes through evidence-driven performance improvement. The JTS vision is that every Soldier, Sailor, Airman and Marine injured on the battlefield or in any theatre of operations will be provided with the optimum chance for survival and maximum potential for functional recovery. It covers Joint Clinical Practice Guidelines, the US military DoD Trauma Registry with three subordinate clinical domains: TCCC, En-Route Combat Casualty Care (ERCCC), and Surgical Combat Casualty Care (SCCC).

Learning Activity 9.1   Chains of Care – Suggested Answers

Common features in all the 'chains of care' are as follows: *a 'Chain of care' image, incremental increases in clinical capability, bystander first aid, stabilisation units, hospitals and ambulance transport.*

Differences are as follows: *inclusion of non-trauma emergencies, rehabilitation and recovery as a final clinical function, identification of specific health professionals and their competencies, a command and control function.*

Is anything missing? *Possible observations: nuances of providing emergency care for obstetric and paediatric patients, no mention of psychological and social health services, trauma registries, governance/oversight as a function of command and control.*

Case Study: Learning Activity 9.2 – Trauma Registries

The US military 'Joint Trauma System' (JTS) that is underpinned by the US 'Joint Theatre Trauma Registry' (JTTR) is widely cited as the best example of the implementation of a whole system approach to the care of trauma casualties. The paper by Spott et al

(continued)

Case Study: Learning Activity 9.2   Continued

summarises the evolution of the JTS. The JTS has been credited with giving US military casualties the highest chance of survival from any war. These outcomes demonstrate the clinical opportunities associated with the successful implementation of an integrated JTS. A selection of the many academic publications resulting from the US JTS is at: https://jts.health.mil/index.cfm/documents/publications

Without implying criticism of the immense success of the US military JTS, you may wish to consider the following questions after reading the paper: Why did it take from 1996 to 2002 to establish a demonstration project for a trauma registry? Why did it take from 2002 to 2006 before a Director of the JTS was appointed? Why did it take until 2010 to broaden the scope of the JTS from supporting medical operations in the Middle East to supporting all US deployed forces?

The second pair of papers describes the challenges associated with the capture of data for a trauma registry in Tanzania and South Africa, respectively. The first paper highlights the low rate of completion of clinical data for each patient including key information about mechanism of injury and vital signs. The authors suggest that a combination of limited infrastructure, low staffing, and shortage of supplies might be associated with poor compliance with basic data entry into the trauma registry. The second paper is a wider literature review of papers that describe the operation of trauma registries in low- and middle-income countries (LMICs). The paper also highlighted the problems of missing data from clinical fields in trauma registries, variation in the data fields between different trauma systems, and dissemination of findings to improve clinical performance. It is possible for the value of trauma registries in LMICs to be improved with greater standardisation to the WHO dataset, better training, digitally supported data collection, and better feedback loops between clinical evidence derived from the registry and the stakeholders within the trauma system.

NOTES

1. This section of the Health Chapter of the Sphere Handbook also includes the action: ensure timely access to mental health services and psychosocial support. Mental health will be covered in Chapter 13 of this book.

2. Committee on Tactical Combat Casualty Care (CoTCCC). https://jts.health.mil/index.cfm/committees/cotccc.

3. First Aid in Armed Conflicts and Other Situations of Violence. https://www.icrc.org/en/publication/0870-first-aid-armed-conflicts-and-other-situations-violence.

4. Behaviour in Combat: Code of Conduct for Combatants and First Aid Manual. https://www.icrc.org/en/publication/0526-behaviour-combat-code-conduct-combatants-and-first-aid-manual.

5. Major Incident Medical Management and Support. Advanced Life Support Group. Available at https://www.alsg.org/home/.

6. Strengthening rehabilitation in health emergency preparedness, response and resilience: policy brief. Available at https://www.who.int/publications/i/item/9789240073432.

REFERENCES

1. Thompson, F. (2024). Emergency healthcare in crisis. *Bull World Health Organ* 102: 5–6. http://dx.doi.org/10.2471/BLT.24.020124.

2. Werner, K., Kak, M., Herbst, C.H., and Lin, T.K. (2023). Emergency care in post-conflict settings: a systematic literature review. *BMC Emergency Medicine* 23 (1): 37. https://doi.org/10.1186/s12873-023-00775-0.

3. Chatfield-Ball, C., Boyle, P., Autier, P. et al. (2015). Lessons learned from the casualties of war: battlefield medicine and its implication for global trauma care. *Journal of the Royal Society of Medicine* 108 (3): 93–100. https://doi.org/10.1177/0141076815570923.

4. IFRC (2020). International First Aid, Resuscitation and Education Guidelines. International Federation of Red Cross and Red Crescent Societies. https://www.ifrc.org/document/international-first-aid-resuscitation-and-education-guidelines (accessed 3 March 2025).

5. WHO (2025). Interagency Integrated Triage Tool. https://www.who.int/publications/m/item/IITT (accessed 3 March 2025).

6. ICRC (1998). *Hospitals for War-Wounded: A Practical Guide for Setting Up and Running a Surgical Hospital in an Area of Armed Conflict*. Geneva: ICRC. https://www.icrc.org/en/publication/0714-hospitals-war-wounded-practical-guide-setting-and-running-surgical-hospital-area (accessed 3 March 2025).

7. WHO. *Trauma Resuscitation Algorithm*. https://cdn.who.int/media/docs/default-source/integrated-health-services-(ihs)/csy/rad/trauma-algorithm.pdf?sfvrsn=2cefdfd_4 (accessed 3 March 2025).

8. WHO (2016). *Trauma Care Checklist*. https://www.who.int/publications/i/item/trauma-care-checklist (accessed 3 March 2025).

9. WHO (2020). *Medical Emergency Checklist*. https://www.who.int/publications/i/item/who-medical-emergency-checklist (accessed 3 March 2025).

10. Allied Joint Doctrine for Medical Support (2019). AJP 4.10(C) NATO Sep 2019. Lexicon Page Lex-5. https://www.coemed.org/files/stanags/01_AJP/AJP-4.10_EDC_V1_E_2228.pdf (accessed 3 March 2025).

11. WHO. *Rehabilitation*. https://www.who.int/health-topics/rehabilitation#tab=tab_1 (accessed 3 March 2025).

12. Humanity and Inclusion (2020). Early Rehabilitation in Conflicts and Disasters. https://www.hi.org/en/early-rehabilitation-in-conflicts-and-disasters (accessed 3 March 2025).

13. WHO (2023). *Clinical Registry Concept Note*. Geneva: WHO. https://www.who.int/publications/m/item/who-clinical-registry (accessed 3 March 2025).

14. WHO. *Standardized Clinical Form*. Geneva: WHO. https://www.who.int/publications/i/item/who-standardized-clinical-form# (accessed 3 March 2025).

CHAPTER 10

War, Communicable Disease, and Health Security

Gemma Bowsher and Martin Bricknell

Centre for Conflict and Health Security, King's College London, London, UK

Abstract

The aim of this chapter is to examine the relationships between war, communicable disease, and global health security (GHS). War has been the causative factor in the outbreak of many disease epidemics over history. War can disrupt immunisation programmes, break down herd immunity, and erode essential public health safeguards, with the resultant increased risk of outbreaks. This chapter will summarise the major communicable diseases that need to be prevented, detected, and controlled during war and other humanitarian emergencies. The chapter will close by re-considering the topic, GHS from Chapter 7, and the response of national and international actors in protecting the world from catastrophic outbreaks of infectious disease.

Keywords: communicable disease, expanded programme of immunisation, surveillance, outbreak management, global health security

Handbook of Global Health, Security, and War, First Edition. Edited by Martin Bricknell and Richard Sullivan.
© 2025 John Wiley & Sons Ltd. Published 2025 by John Wiley & Sons Ltd.

KEY LEARNING OUTCOMES

By studying this chapter, the reader will be able to:

- Describe how conflict has affected the incidence of infectious disease across history
- Summarise the key principles for the prevention, detection, and control of outbreaks of infectious disease in disasters and other emergencies
- Refresh the concepts underpinning the term 'global health security' (GHS)

INTRODUCTION

Chapter 1 introduced **public health** and **global health** as the domains of technical knowledge for the prevention of disease, the protection of health, and the promotion of healthy lifestyles for human, national and global security. Public health practitioners achieve this at the community level through immunisation campaigns, health education, environmental health, and other community and societal efforts. Global health applies these concepts at the level of international relations. Chapter 2 placed health in the perspective of security and introduced the concepts of **global health security (**GHS) and **one health**. Chapter 3 discussed the impact of conflict on health and health services, showing that secondary and tertiary impacts can disrupt public health programmes and the societal determinants of health such as shelter, water, sanitation, and food supplies. Chapter 4 discussed the impact of conflict on the displacement and migration of populations, and Chapter 5 included epidemic threats (communicable diseases) within the **CBRNE3T** (**c**hemical, **b**iological, **r**adiological, **n**uclear (CBRN), **e**xplosive, **e**ndemic, **e**nvironmental, and non-battle **t**rauma) classification of threats to health during conflict. Chapter 7 provided a summary of the concept of GHS.

This chapter is based on Section 2.1 Communicable Disease of the Health Chapter in the Sphere Handbook on pages 311–322. The key areas for action for communicable diseases during a humanitarian emergency are to:

- Ensure people have access to healthcare and information to prevent communicable diseases
- Establish surveillance and reporting systems to provide early outbreak detection and early response
- Ensure people have access to effective diagnosis and treatment for infectious diseases that contribute most significantly to morbidity and mortality
- Ensure outbreaks are adequately prepared for and controlled in a timely and effective manner

Communicable disease risks and mitigations will also be considered in other chapters. HIV and sexually transmitted diseases will be considered in the section on reproductive health in Chapter 10 Maternal and Child Health. Chapter 10 will also cover the role of childhood immunisation programmes for the protection of children from communicable diseases. Please undertake Learning Activity 10.1 to introduce you to the links between war and epidemics.

Learning Activity 10.1   War and Epidemics

Please watch the YouTube video for a short summary of significant pandemics in global history: The Most Destructive Pandemics and Epidemics in Human History – https://www.youtube.com/watch?v=hD8Hfj_eYZ0

Using Google and other online resources, create a timeline/list of major epidemics associated with war in human history.

You may wish to use the following additional resources to assist in your analysis:

Kaniewski, D. and Marriner, N. (2020). Conflicts and the spread of plagues in pre-industrial Europe. *Humanities and Social Sciences Communications* 162 (7): 1–10. https://doi.org/10.1057/s41599-020-00661-1.

Roy, K, and Ray, S. (2018). War and epidemics: a chronicle of infectious diseases. *Journal of Marine Medical Society* 20 (1): 50–54. https://www.researchgate.net/publication/326288278_War_and_epidemics_A_chronicle_of_infectious_diseases/fulltext/5b4415efa6f dcc6619140335/War-and-epidemics-A-chronicle-of-infectious-diseases.pdf?origin=publication_detail&_tp=eyJjb250ZXh0I jp7ImZpcnN0UGFnZSI6InB1YmxpY2F0aW9uIiwicGFnZSI6InB1YmxpY2F 0aW9uRG93bmxvYWQiLCJwcmV2aW91c1BhZ2UiOiJwdWJsaWNhdGlvbiJ9 fQ&__cf_chl_tk=GWHZQczTL7F4p0W4tsmrtt_UQ5.826QwhjEmm3seUCY-1750663936-1.0.1.1-aU0YiC1NhtYsQd6KglS0VljVpSOjLwll40Y2soLUkD4.

Councell, CE. (1941). War and infectious disease. *Public Health Reports* 56 (12): 547–573. https://doi.org/10.2307/4583663.

Suggested answers are at the end of the chapter.

COMMUNICABLE DISEASE THREATS IN HUMANITARIAN EMERGENCIES

As shown in Learning Activity 10.1, the interrelationships between war and infectious disease are well known. Prior to the introduction of immunisation and antibiotics, disease was the primary cause of death amongst armies. Conflict also promotes the conditions for outbreaks of infectious diseases amongst civilians often causing a death toll that exceeds the number of deaths from physical trauma. The breakdown of public health systems, the mass movement of displaced populations, poor shelter and overcrowding, disruption of water and food supplies, and destruction of sanitation all create the conditions for rapid transmission of infectious diseases [1]. A review of academic literature on the impact of recent conflicts on infectious diseases confirmed this list, and the importance of both general preparedness and response strategies for infectious disease outbreaks and measures to protect and control against specific diseases (such as HIV, cholera, acute respiratory diseases, tuberculosis, poliomyelitis, malaria, leishmaniasis, measles, dengue, diphtheria, and acute bacterial meningitis) [2].

Infectious diseases can be divided by type of causative organism (virus, bacteria, fungus, parasite) or routes of infection (which may be more useful when considering methods of control). The most common routes of transmission are from food/water (ingestion) and airborne (inhalation). Vector-borne diseases require another animal to transmit the disease via a bite, usually insects. Bloodborne diseases are transmitted through contact with the blood of the infected person. Some infective agents can persist in the environment by contaminating surfaces and being transmitted by touch to broken skin or to the mouth/nose. Sexually transmitted diseases are transmitted during sexual acts. Finally, the healthcare setting is a high-risk environment because infected patients may expose other patients, visitors, or healthcare workers to any of these routes with the added risk of antimicrobial resistance in the infective agent. Table 10.1 shows a list of some diseases at risk of causing outbreaks during a humanitarian emergency categorised by route of transmission (Table 10.1).

Whilst there may be public health interventions that apply to a specific infectious disease (e.g. immunisation, chlorination of water supplies), it is necessary to apply a 'whole of society approach' to manage the risk of infectious disease outbreaks developing into epidemics because all members of a community need to contribute to breaking the chain of transmission. This includes community engagement, community empowerment, and community receptiveness to public health and social measures that might constrain normal social activities. The World Health Organization (WHO) handbook for managing epidemics provides an excellent summary on the overall management of an outbreak and key facts about the diseases most at risk of causing an epidemic [4]. The four 'operational stages' are summarised below:

1. **Prevent and Prepare**: the application of preventive measures and preparation of the response to outbreaks.
2. **Respond**: get ready and contain: the detection and containment of an outbreak to try to break transmission.
3. **Respond**: control/reduce transmission and mitigate the impact: escalation of public health measures to wider communities and non-health measures to mitigate the impact of the outbreak (e.g. economic support).
4. **Recover**: scale down and sustain control measures, elimination of the risk of resurgence: the de-escalation of the response whilst ensuring that the cause of the outbreak can be eradicated.

TABLE 10.1 Classification of infectious diseases by route of transmission.

Route	Disease
Food/water	Cholera, hepatitis A and E, polio, typhoid, Shigella, *E. coli*
Airborne	Measles, meningococcal meningitis, pneumonia, tuberculosis, diphtheria, pertussis, influenza, plague
Vector borne	Malaria, typhus, yellow fever, dengue, Crimean–Congo haemorrhagic fever, plague
Bloodborne	Hepatitis, HIV
Surface contact	Ebola, Lassa fever
Sexually transmission	Syphilis, gonorrhoea, HIV, hepatitis B
Healthcare	'All of the above', anti-microbial-resistant (AMR) organisms

Source: Modified from [3].

These operational stages include ensuring that affected populations can access safe and effective clinical care alongside protecting healthcare workers from the risk of transmission of the disease. It is also important to maintain other essential health services (e.g. emergency services and maternal and child healthcare) during the outbreak. Specific information about the clinical management and public health control measures for individual communicable diseases can usually be found from the websites of the WHO and national public health organizations such as the US Centers for Disease Control and Prevention and the UK Health Security Agency (the websites are listed at the end of this chapter).

NON-HEALTH PREVENTION OF DISEASE OUTBREAKS

The non-health chapters of the Sphere Handbook contain vital standards for the prevention of outbreaks of infectious diseases. The Water Supply, Sanitation, and Hygiene Promotion (WASH) chapter has six sections that cover hygiene promotion, water supply, excreta management, vector control, solid waste management, and WASH in disease outbreaks and healthcare settings. These emphasise the importance of environmental health and sanitary engineers in reducing the risks of diseases transmitted by the oral–faecal route and the critical importance of clean, safe water. The section on vector control covers measures to prevent insect-borne diseases, especially those transmitted by flies and mosquitos. The chapter on Shelter and Settlement describes how planning can reduce disease transmission amongst communities and setting minimum standards can prevent transmission of diseases due to overcrowding (e.g. respiratory diseases). These chapters also provide sources of reference for planning data and other technical instructions for WASH and public health engineering.

SURVEILLANCE, DETECTION, AND CONTROL OF OUTBREAKS OF COMMUNICABLE DISEASES

An outbreak of a disease can be defined when the incidence (number of new cases during a specified time period for a population at risk) exceeds the expected background incidence. This varies according to the disease. Although this definition is framed in regard to communicable diseases, this definition can apply to any disease (such as an exposure to an environmental chemical). The investigation of an outbreak is founded upon the basic epidemiological questions: **What** is the disease (which requires a 'case definition'), **who** are affected, **where** have they been infected, and over what **time** period have the infections occurred? Collecting data based on these parameters provides answers to **how** they were infected, what **response** is required, and how to **communicate** and **implement** the response within affected communities. These principles apply to all outbreaks of disease; however, the risk of an outbreak and the detection and response to an outbreak are likely to be more complicated in a fragile or conflict-affected population compared to well-resourced and stable communities.

The operational stages described in Section 2 of this chapter highlight the importance of routine health surveillance and disease reporting as a baseline task for health systems. The Sphere Handbook describes the requirement for disease Early Warning,

Alert, and Response (EWAR) mechanisms for priority diseases and events that may require an immediate response.[1] The International Health Regulations (IHR) 2005 lists four diseases that must be notified by national authorities (smallpox, poliomyelitis caused by wild-type poliovirus, a new subtype of human influenza, and severe acute respiratory syndrome (SARS)); and other diseases that should be notified such as cholera, pneumonic plague, yellow fever, viral haemorrhagic fever, West Nile fever, and other biological, chemical, or radiological events that meet the criteria of being at risk of causing a serious public health emergency, is unusual or unexpected, has a risk of international spread, or may require control by restrictions on international travel or trade.

The first phase of response after the detection of an outbreak is to form an Outbreak Control Team (OCT). The role of an OCT is to:

- determine if an outbreak has occurred,
- determine the risk to the health of the population at risk,
- develop a plan to contain the outbreak,
- determine who needs to be informed, and
- to co-ordinate the implementation of the response.

National and international organisational policies are likely to specify the processes and procedures to be followed in the management of a disease outbreak. Examples include the WHO Field Manual for Communicable Disease Control in Emergencies [4], the UN High Commission for Refugees guidance on epidemic preparedness and response in refugee camp settings [5], and the UK operational guidance for communicable disease outbreak management [6].

The global approach to outbreak control is based on the IHR 2005 [7]. The IHR provides a framework of international law that describes the rights and obligations of countries in responding to public health events and emergencies which have the potential to cross international borders. These have been ratified by the 194 member states of the World Health Assembly. These regulations cover the obligation of countries to notify the WHO of incidents which might meet the criteria to be a 'public health event of international concern' (PHEIC) based on a decision tree in Annex 2 of the IHR. Since 2007, the WHO has declared PHEICs in response to the following outbreaks: 2009 H1N1 swine flu, 2014 rise in cases of wild polio, 2014–2016 West African outbreak of Ebola, 2016 Zika virus outbreak, 2018–2019 Ebola outbreak in the Democratic Republic of Congo, 2019–2023 COVID-19 pandemic, and 2022 monkeypox outbreak. The WHO initiated an Intergovernmental Negotiating Body to develop a Pandemic Agreement as an update to the IHR in 2021. The global response and subsequent coordination work after the COVID-19 pandemic will be discussed in Chapter 16.

(GLOBAL) HEALTH SECURITY

The implementation of IHR 2005 requires countries to have eight core capacities:

1. National legislation, policy, and financing
2. Coordination and national focal point communications

3. Surveillance
4. Response
5. Preparedness
6. Risk communication
7. Human resources
8. Laboratory services

The WHO established an IHR Monitoring Framework and an IHR Monitoring Tool to assist states to develop their IHR core capabilities. However, experience during the response to the PHEICs of the second decade of the 21st century and national reporting showed weaknesses in the global capacity to implement the IHRs [8]. Concurrently, there was increasing recognition that threats from communicable diseases to public health could have impacts beyond health to become a direct threat to national security. Thus, as described in Chapter 2, health threats became listed within national security risk registers and the term 'global health security' emerged to frame health security as a public good within the global commons [9]. Chapter 7 described how GHS became a phrase to increase governmental and societal awareness of the potential consequences of health threats on national and global security.

The WHO defines global public health security as:

'the activities required, both proactive and reactive, to minimize the danger and impact of acute public health events that endanger people's health across geographical regions and international boundaries' [10].

The term 'health security' features prominently in various international fora,[2] international organisations[3], and countries' health strategies [11, 12]. The scope of the term 'health security' has been extended from infectious disease to include all biological threats, including threats to plant and animal health, and the threat from chemical and biological weapons. This has led to the emergence of the term 'One Health' to reflect the interdependence of health for humans, domestic and wild animals, plants, and wider biological ecosystems in the prevention, detection, response, and management of disease risks [13]. This also widens the scientific and professional disciplines with a stake in GHS and the need for GHS to be embedded within Universal Health Care as part of health emergency planning [14].

NON-HEALTH IMPACTS OF HEALTH SECURITY CRISES

Many commentators consider the COVID-19 pandemic to be the archetypal event that exposed national and global weaknesses in the management of an entirely predictable health security risk. It demonstrated the non-health risks and impacts of a health crisis on all dimensions of national and international security. Please undertake Learning Activity 10.2 to use a framework to explore these interdependencies.

Learning Activity 10.2   Case Study – The COVID-19 Pandemic Through a Security Lens

Chapter 2 described dimensions of national security using the acronym MIDFIELD (military, information, diplomatic, financial, intelligence, economic, legal, and development). Using the table below (Table 10.2), add examples of how the COVID-19 pandemic affected each dimension. The following sources may assist with this task.

Watch: A look back at the COVID-19 pandemic | COVID-19 Special. Available at `https://www.youtube.com/watch?v=1B9Koo7fHE4`

Consider reviewing the following information sources:

European Health Observatory. COVID-19 Health System Response Monitor (HSRM): `https://eurohealthobservatory.who.int/monitors/hsrm/`

Baciu, C. (2021). Beyond the emergency *problematique*: how do security IOs respond to crises—a case study of NATO response to COVID-19. *Journal of Transatlantic Studies* 19: 261–281. https://doi.org/10.1057/s42738-021-00079-w.

TABLE 10.2   Non-health dimensions of the COVID-19 pandemic as a security crisis – example answers.

Dimension	Impact of COVID-19
Military	
Information	
Diplomatic	
Financial	
Intelligence	
Economic	
Legal	
Development	

LOOKING FORWARD

This chapter has provided an overview to communicable diseases and how these can be mitigated during a humanitarian emergency. The chapter closed by considering threats to health as a risk to security and the emergence of the 'GHS' perspective. The next chapter will consider maternal and child health in the context of humanitarian emergencies. It will also cover the role of routine childhood immunisation programmes for the prevention of communicable disease.

SOURCES AND RESOURCES

Suggested Internet search terms are as follows: 'communicable disease humanitarian'; 'biosecurity'; and 'global health security',

Suggested websites and online sources for further information:

International/National websites:
World Health Organization:

Global Health Emergencies – `https://www.who.int/emergencies/overview`
Health Security – `https://www.who.int/health-topics/health-security#tab=tab_1`
Outbreak toolkit – `https://www.who.int/emergencies/outbreak-toolkit`
US Centre for Disease Control – `https://www.cdc.gov/index.htm`
UK Health Security Agency – `https://www.gov.uk/government/organisations/uk-health-security-agency`

Reference 'Books'

UK Green Book – Immunisation against infectious disease `https://www.gov.uk/government/collections/immunisation-against-infectious-disease-the-green-book`
US Control of Communicable Diseases Manual – `https://www.apha.org/publications/published-books/ccdm`

Learning Activity 10.1 Suggested Answers

Refer to the timeline within the UK biosecurity strategy – license from visual capitalist – `https://www.visualcapitalist.com/history-of-pandemics-deadliest/`

Learning Activity 10.2 Case Study – The COVID-19 Pandemic Through a Security Lens – Suggested Answers (Table 10.3)

TABLE 10.3 Non-health dimensions of the COVID-19 pandemic as a security crisis – example answers.

Dimension	Impact of COVID-19
Military	Outbreaks in military bases and ships, non-availability of personnel due to family care, employment of armed forces to support civilian response, international military–military COVID-19 assistance
Information	'Dis-information', challenges of public communication
Diplomatic	New alliances based on COVID-19 support, vaccine diplomacy
Financial	Increased exposure to financial crime, fraud and corruption in contracting
Intelligence	Barriers to open information sharing, industrial espionage, intelligence applied to domestic populations
Economic	Huge economic hit, extension of government borrowing, risk to jobs and livelihoods
Legal	Weakening of democratic safeguards, extension of government powers on personal behaviours
Development	Reduction in global development assistance funding, reduced access to vulnerable populations due to travel restrictions, decrease in progress towards SDGs

NOTES

1. Sphere Handbook. Health Systems Standard 1.5. Page 308 and Communicable disease standard 2.1.2. Page 314.
2. For example, the Global Health Security Agenda. Available at `https://globalhealthsecurityagenda.org/` and the Global Health Security Initiative. Available at `https://ghsi.ca/`.
3. For example, EU Global Health Strategy. Available at `https://health.ec.europa.eu/internationalcooperation/global-health_en#global-health-security-initiative`.

REFERENCES

1. Connolly, M.A. and Heymann, D.L. (2002). Deadly comrades: war and infectious diseases. *The Lancet* 360: s23–s24. `https://doi.org/10.1016/S0140-6736(02)11807-1`.
2. Marou, V., Vardavas, C.I., Aslanoglou, K. et al. (2024). The impact of conflict on infectious disease: a systematic literature review. *Conflict and Health* 18 (1): 27. `https://doi.org/10.1186/s13031-023-00568-z`.
3. WHO (2023). *Managing Epidemics: Key Facts About Major Deadly Diseases*, 2e. Geneva: WHO. `https://www.who.int/publications/i/item/9789240083196`.
4. WHO (2005). *Communicable Disease Control in Emergencies: A Field Manual*. World Health Organization. `https://www.who.int/publications/i/item/communicable-disease-control-in-emergencies-a-field-manual` (accessed 29 March 2025).
5. UNHCR (2011). Epidemic Preparedness and Response in Refugee Camp Settings. Guidance for Public Health Officers. UNHCR. `https://www.unhcr.org/uk/media/epidemic-preparednes-and-response-refugee-camp-settings-guidance-public-health-officers` (accessed 29 March 2025).
6. GOV.UK (2023). *Communicable Disease Outbreak Management: Operational Guidance*. UK Health Security Agency. `https://www.gov.uk/government/publications/communicable-disease-outbreak-management-operational-guidance` (accessed 29 March 2025).
7. WHO (2005). *International Health Regulations*. World Health Organization. `https://www.who.int/health-topics/international-health-regulations#tab=tab_1` (accessed 29 March 2025).
8. Gostin, L.O. and Katz, R. (2016). The international health regulations: the governing framework for global health security. *The Milbank Quarterly* 94 (2): 264–313. `https://doi.org/10.1111/1468-0009.12186`.
9. McCoy, D., Roberts, S., Daoudi, S., and Kennedy, J. (2023). Global health security and the health-security nexus: principles, politics and praxis. *BMJ Global Health* 8: e013067. `https://doi.org/10.1136/bmjgh-2023-013067`.
10. WHO. *Health Security*. Geneva: WHO. `https://www.who.int/health-topics/health-security#tab=tab_1` (accessed 29 March 2025).
11. GOV.UK (2023). UK Biological Security Strategy. London: Cabinet office. `https://www.gov.uk/government/publications/uk-biological-security-strategy` (accessed 29 March 2025).

12. ASPR (2022). *US National Biodefense Strategy*. White House. `https://aspr.hhs.gov/biodefense/Pages/default.aspx` (accessed 29 March 2025).

13. Lefrançois, T., Malvy, D., Atlani-Duault, L. et al. (2023). After 2 years of the COVID-19 pandemic, translating One Health into action is urgent. *The Lancet* 401 (10378): 789–794. `https://doi.org/10.1016/S0140-6736(22)01840-2`.

14. Kamradt-Scott, A., Teo, Y.Y., and Katz, R. (2022). Singapore statement on global health security. *BMJ Global Health* 7: e009949. `https://doi.org/10.1136/bmjgh-2022-009949`.

CHAPTER 11

War and Maternal and Child Health

Lucy Singh[1], Peter von Dadelszen[1] and Martin Bricknell[2]

[1] Department of Women & Children's Health, School of Life Course & Population Sciences, King's College London, London, UK

[2] Centre for Conflict and Health Security, King's College London, London, UK

Abstract

The aim of this chapter is to review how war affects maternal and child health and the essential clinical services needed to meet the needs of these patients. This chapter will start by considering essential maternity care to detect and treat emergencies during pregnancy and childbirth. It will then look at risks to the health of newborns, babies, and children, particularly linking to the risk of contracting the communicable diseases described in Chapter 10. It will close by considering conflict-related sexual violence (CRSV) as a weapon of war and the impact on affected women.

Keywords: maternal health, child health, childhood immunisation, gender-based violence

Handbook of Global Health, Security, and War, First Edition. Edited by Martin Bricknell and Richard Sullivan.
© 2025 John Wiley & Sons Ltd. Published 2025 by John Wiley & Sons Ltd.

KEY LEARNING OUTCOMES

By studying this chapter, the reader will be able to:

- Describe the impacts of conflict on sexual, reproductive, maternal, newborn, and child health
- Outline the particular risks to women and children during conflict and other humanitarian emergencies
- Describe the key principles of health service provision for sexual, reproductive, maternal, newborn, and child health in conflict-affected populations

---

INTRODUCTION

Chapter 3 showed how the impact of war on health affects many more civilians than military personnel engaged in direct combat. Although civilians often attempt to flee from the front lines, the threats to health from displacement (primarily communicable diseases and mental ill-health), the disruption of health services, and the tertiary impacts of war on the determinants of health will result in a substantial increase in morbidity and mortality amongst civilians. These secondary and tertiary impacts disproportionately affect women and children compared with male civilians. A literature review by Garry and Checchi on the impact of armed conflict and public health showed that armed conflict can have catastrophic effects on the health of infants, children, and women because of their vulnerabilities to general health threats caused by conflict and also because of their specific risk of trafficking, recruitment of **child soldiers**, and **gender-based violence** (GBV). The mental health consequences of conflict can endure across a life course, and there is emerging evidence of inter-generational effects of war on health including environmental contamination (nuclear and chemical agents) from remnants of war causing birth defects, maternal malnutrition affecting foetal and postnatal growth and development, and psychological consequences of war affecting child development and learned adult behaviour [1].

This chapter is based upon Section 2.2 Child Health and Section 2.3 Sexual and Reproductive Health (SRH) of the Health Chapter in the *Sphere Handbook* at pages 335–339. The key standards for Child Health and SRH care during a humanitarian emergency are

- Children aged six months to 15 years have immunity against disease and access to routine Expanded Programme on Immunization (EPI) services during crises (links to Chapter 10 Communicable Disease).
- Children have access to priority healthcare that addresses the major causes of newborn and childhood morbidity and mortality.
- People have access to healthcare and family planning that prevents excessive maternal and newborn morbidity and mortality.

- People have access to healthcare that is safe and responds to the needs of survivors of sexual violence.
- People have access to healthcare that prevents transmission and reduces morbidity and mortality due to human immunodeficiency virus (HIV) (links to Chapter 10 Communicable Disease).

The chapter on Food Security and Nutrition in the Sphere Handbook also contains important standards for the management of malnutrition and the feeding of infants and young children.

Please undertake Learning Activity 11.1 to further understand the impact of war on women and children.

Learning Activity 11.1   Incidence and Consequence of War on Women and Children

Watch the YouTube video: War on Children Campaign. Save the Children. https://www.youtube.com/watch?v=5KTVEMVS_X0

Read the following academic papers:

Bendavid, E., Boerma, T., Akseer, N. et al. (2021). The effects of armed conflict on the health of women and children. *The Lancet* 397 (10273): 522–532. https://doi.org/10.1016/S0140-6736(21)00131-8.

Amberg, F., Chansa, C., Niangaly, H. et al. (2023). Examining the relationship between armed conflict and coverage of maternal and child health services in 35 countries in sub-Saharan Africa: a geospatial analysis. *The Lancet Global Health* 11 (6): e843–e853. https://www.thelancet.com/journals/langlo/article/PIIS2214-109X(23)00152-3/fulltext

How do the video and the academic evidence of the impact of war on women and children make you feel?

The disruption caused by conflict and war can have severe effects on the provision of SRH services. The Inter-Agency Working Group on Reproductive Health in Crises sponsors the Inter-Agency Field Manual on Reproductive Health in Humanitarian Settings and the Minimum Initial Service Package for SRH in Crisis Situations (MISP) [2]. The MISP is a set of priority and lifesaving SRH services and activities to be implemented at the onset of every humanitarian emergency to prevent excess SRH-related morbidity and mortality. The objectives cover:

- system leadership,
- prevention and response to sexual violence,
- prevention and treatment of sexually transmitted infections (STIs),
- prevention of maternal and newborn morbidity and mortality, and
- prevention of unintended pregnancies.

Clinical SRH services cover family planning, antenatal care, care at the time of delivery, and postnatal care for women and babies. The section 'Community Sexual and Reproductive Health' of this chapter will cover the community-based services for SRH usually provided by nurses, midwives, and doctors working in community health clinics. The section 'Antenatal, Intrapartum, and Postnatal Care' will cover hospital-provided antenatal, intrapartum (during delivery) and postpartum care, and the section 'Newborn Care' will cover care of the newborn. The Section 'Conflict-Related Sexual Violence' will cover conflict-related sexual violence (CRSV) and GBV. SRH services should respect the cultural backgrounds and religious beliefs of both the supported community and the host community, but should also reflect the global consensus on human rights, particularly the rights of women to choices regarding their own health. SRH and child health services must be sensitive to the psychological needs and understanding of children, adolescents, young adults, and persons with disabilities, acknowledging their sexual orientation and gender identity.

The provision of SRH and child health services can be considered as a layered 'chain of care' in the same way as discussed for trauma services in Chapter 9. This is illustrated in Figure 11.1. There are considered to be three potential delays in maternal care: delay in recognising the need to seek health care at the household level; delay in reaching health care due to distance to health facilities, lack of transport, and poor quality of routes; and delay in receiving adequate healthcare due to poor facilities, lack of supplies, and lack of competent health professionals. The transport problem can occur from household to primary care (transport 1) and from primary care to hospital care (transport 2), resulting in four critical connection points to the continuity of care: between stages of pregnancy, between families and healthcare workers, between health facilities, and between multiple care-seeking journeys [3]. These challenges are compounded in conflict settings where the health system is fragile and fragmented. Humanitarian and medical personnel providing healthcare are protected under International Humanitarian Law under UN Security Council Resolution (UNSCR) 2286. Despite this, there continue to be attacks involving healthcare facilities in conflict settings resulting in the loss of infrastructure, services, and skilled health personnel. In many conflict-affected settings, pregnant and postpartum women may have limited autonomy of decision-making (e.g. leaving the home in an emergency

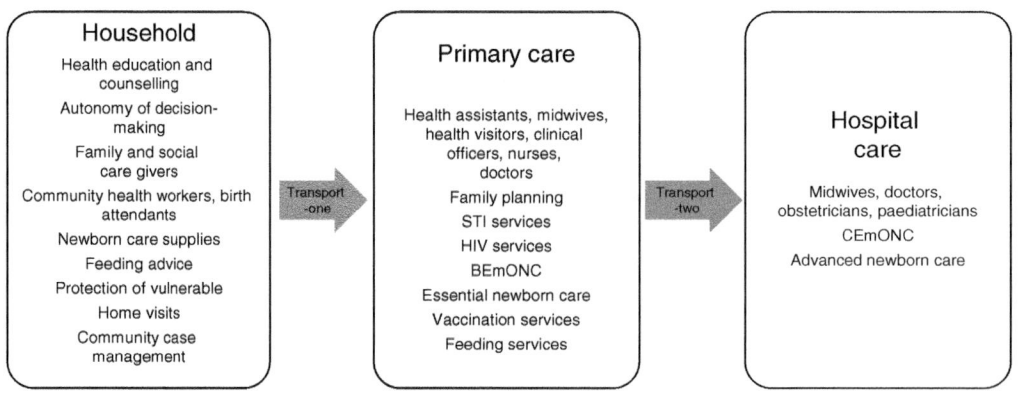

Sexually transmitted infection - STI
Basic emergency obstetric and newborn care – BEmONC
Comprehensive emergency obstetric and newborn care - CEmONC

FIGURE 11.1   Chain of care: maternal and child health.

without explicit male permission) that can further compound the delays. Delays in accessing timely, quality maternal and child health services increase morbidity and mortality.

COMMUNITY SEXUAL AND REPRODUCTIVE HEALTH

An important aspect of SRH clinical services is the provision of menstrual health, family planning advice, and contraceptive services. These services should be available to individuals across the life course, tailored according to the age, needs, social and cultural values of individuals accessing the services. Contraceptives should be available to enable individuals to make their own choices about pregnancy and to reduce the risk of STIs. The MISP specifies that even in the acute phase of a conflict, services should provide a range of methods for regular and emergency contraception. Community-based SRH services should also include referral of women in the event of pregnancy to midwifery, to safe abortion services (or post-abortion care as a minimum where abortion is illegal), and sterilisation services (e.g. vasectomy). More information on family planning services, including a list of types of contraception, is available in the World Health Organization (WHO) Family Planning Handbook [4].

The prevention of HIV and other STIs is an essential element of SRH services. STIs are those diseases that are transmitted through sexual activity and can infect the genitals, the area around the genitalia, the anus, and the mouth. These can be caused by bacteria (e.g. chancroid, chlamydia, gonorrhoea, and syphilis), viruses (e.g. herpes, hepatitis B (HepB), human papillomavirus (HPV), HIV), and parasites (trichomoniasis). These can be prevented by barrier methods of contraception (condoms), vaccination against HepB and HPV, or pre-exposure/post-exposure prophylaxis (e.g. HIV). Some STIs can cause early symptoms, such as ulcers, discharge, pain passing urine, and pain during sex. Others can occur without obvious symptoms until significant harm has occurred (e.g. chlamydia, syphilis, and viral infections). SRH for STIs requires community-based education, the provision of post-exposure prophylaxis, and diagnostic and treatment services which may be linked to family planning services. Counselling and provision of STI services should also be provided alongside services for gender-based violence.

Particular care should be taken to include population groups within SRH service provision who are often neglected, such as adolescents. The Adolescent Sexual and Reproductive Health Toolkit for Humanitarian Settings, co-published by Save the Children and the UN Population Fund, provides guidance on the provision of SRH services to adolescent populations affected by conflict [5]. This document emphasises the importance of understanding the risks faced by adolescents of all genders from lack of sex and relationship education, disrupted social settings, sexual exploitation and abuse, and direct sexual violence. These risks may be compounded by social and cultural values that prevent individuals from fulfilling their sexual and reproductive rights. Ideally, providers of SRH services should collaborate with schools and other education settings to enable adolescents to have sufficient health education to understand their own reproductive rights. In practice, this may be challenging with access to education facilities often limited in conflict settings. Other adaptive strategies may include use of mobile clinics, outreach activities in adolescent-friendly settings, and use of peer education.

ANTENATAL, INTRAPARTUM, AND POSTNATAL CARE

Access to good quality antenatal (during pregnancy), intrapartum (during labour and birth), and postnatal (after birth) care is essential to reduce maternal and neonatal death and ill health. A review by Singh NS and others showed variation in the provision of women and child health services in areas of conflict with many barriers to success across the WHO building blocks of health systems. The principal determinant is insecurity that restricts access to health facilities, disincentivises health professionals, destroys infrastructure, and disrupts the logistics for essential supplies and medicines [6].

Basic antenatal and postnatal care may be provided in the community or the home. The World Health Organization recommends that all births take place within the presence of a skilled attendant (a trained midwife, nurse, or doctor) in a facility equipped to manage any obstetric emergencies arising during the birth. Primary care services may be the location for births in uncomplicated pregnancies (usually midwife-led). Secondary care services will provide access to obstetric and neonatal/paediatric care. Referral to secondary care may arise from complications during the pregnancy (e.g. pre-eclampsia) or at the time of delivery.

This chapter will not cover the detailed arrangements of clinical services and clinical practice for the management of women during labour. The WHO publishes multiple resources on care during pregnancy and birth, which are listed at the end of this chapter. This includes the WHO Safe Childbirth Checklist, which provides an aide-memoire for the key decisions for a clinician during childbirth, mirroring the checklists previously discussed in Chapter 8 for trauma services. Similar to the packages of training for trauma, Emergency Obstetrics and Neonatal Care (EmONC) is a widely used brand for the skills training needed for midwives and doctors in the management of intrapartum emergencies [7]. Médecins Sans Frontieres publishes a practical guide for midwives and doctors regarding the management of obstetric emergencies [8].

NEWBORN CARE

In addition to the guidance on the care of mothers during childbirth, it is important that birth attendants, midwives, and doctors are trained in the care of the newborn. This covers the immediate period after delivery and the subsequent days as the mother and child adapt to each other. About half of the under-5 mortality occurs in the newborn period from birth to 28 days. The main causes of death are complications from preterm birth, delivery complications, severe infections, and congenital abnormalities. Many of these deaths are preventable by good obstetric care and good neonatal care. The Newborn Health in Humanitarian Settings Field Guide provides a description of the organisation of health services for newborns [9]. In the immediate post-delivery period, the baby should be kept warm, the mother supported to feed, and infections prevented or rapidly treated. Babies should be monitored to ensure that they gain weight and generally thrive. Inevitably, there are variations in the completeness of adoption of interventions to improve newborn care in humanitarian settings [10].

CHILD HEALTH AND PROTECTION

One in six children live in a conflict setting. For children whose mother dies when they are ≤42 days, there is a 36-fold increased risk of their child dying within the first six months of life, compared with children whose mother survives, dropping to threefold between 6 and 12 months if the child survives to 6 months. Children whose mother dies when they are ≤1 year bear a 16-fold increased risk of dying during that year [11]. The major causes of death and sickness for children between newborn and age five years are malaria, pneumonia, diarrhoea, HIV, and tuberculosis. Older children are also vulnerable to trauma injuries and wounds from their general environment and specifically explosive remnants of war (landmines and unexploded ordnance). Children may also be affected by the psychological consequences of conflict, a difficult community environment, sexual exploitation, and recruitment as soldiers [12]. Child health services aim to mitigate these impacts through health promotion, immunisation, monitoring and treatment of malnutrition, and diagnosis and treatment of disease, especially infectious disease. The Chapter on Food Security and Nutrition in the Sphere Handbook contains guidance for the response to malnutrition amongst infants and children. Malnutrition is a very significant risk factor for death from infectious diseases. Child health services should have close coordination with education services particularly in the provision of mental health and psychological support, which will be covered in Chapter 13.

Immunisation is the most effective way to prevent vaccine-preventable disease (VPD). This links to the discussion on communicable diseases in Chapter 10. All countries have national vaccination programmes that are initiated close to birth. These are usually based upon the WHO EPI covering, Bacillus Calmette–Guérin (BCG), diphtheria, pertussis, tetanus (DPT), haemophilus influenzae type B (Hib), HepB, polio, measles, rubella, pneumococcal disease (PNC), rotavirus (Rota), HPV, and COVID-19 (for adults). The schedule may include BCG vaccination at birth, DPT, and polio at 6, 10, and 14 weeks, with some countries including Hib, Hep B, PNC, Rota, and meningococcus in the early childhood schedule. Measles, mumps, and rubella can be included at one year and HPV for adolescents. Vaccinations can also be used to prevent other diseases for travellers including hepatitis A, typhoid, cholera, yellow fever, and rabies.

Routine immunisation programmes are frequently disrupted by conflict. In addition to the general effect of conflict on health systems, there are additional impacts on health information, access of vaccination teams to populations, and vaccine distribution chains. A review of vaccine programmes during humanitarian crises suggested that vaccine use during humanitarian crises was insufficient and did not align with the disease burden of affected populations [13]. Preventing outbreaks of VPD through restoration of immunisation programmes is likely to be a high priority for the Health Cluster in a humanitarian emergency. The WHO Vaccination in Humanitarian Emergencies provides a framework for decision-making for vaccination programmes in humanitarian emergencies and a guide to the implementation of a programme [14].

Clinical services for children should recognise that their health needs are different from those of adults. The World Health Organization has sponsored the Integrated Management of Childhood Illness (ICMI) strategy to strengthen the prevention and management of common childhood illnesses through improving health systems, community practices, and the skills and knowledge of healthcare workers. The website provides links to manuals and guidelines for the care of the sick child including the WHO Manual for the health care of children in humanitarian emergencies [15]. At a community level, a community health worker can be trained to identify children with dangerous signs and to refer them to a health facility; to manage dehydration and mild presentations of conditions such as fever, diarrhoea, pneumonia, and malnutrition; and to advise on caring for sick children at home. At the primary care level, the assessment and treatment of the children should be based on the 2022 WHO Pocket Book of Primary Healthcare for Children and Adolescents [16]. A similar pocketbook is available to guide hospital care for children [17].

The protection of vulnerable populations is a central element of the Sphere Handbook and the Humanitarian Charter.[1] Children are a significant proportion of crisis-affected populations and are particularly vulnerable to exploitation if they have been separated from their families. Children with disabilities are at particular risk of neglect. Exploitation can be trafficking for work, recruitment into armed groups, or physical or sexual violence. Conflict and displacement disrupt social order, which can substantially increase the risk of sexual violence against children. Sexual violence is defined as any form of sexual activity with a child by an adult or another child with power over the child.

In addition to the *Sphere Handbook*, the Alliance for Child Protection in Humanitarian Action has published the Child Protection Minimum Standards (CPMS) in order to establish common principles and to strengthen coordination between those working in child protection during humanitarian crises [18]. These are based upon the UN Convention on the Rights of a Child, augmented by the protection principles from the Sphere Charter, and tailored to the specific requirements of children. All organisations and people working in the humanitarian sector, especially those with a remit to care for children and young people, are encouraged to adhere to the CPMS. Maternal and child health services in humanitarian and conflict-affected settings should specifically consider how they can meet the needs of, and contribute to the protection of, vulnerable populations through cross-sectoral engagement.

CONFLICT-RELATED SEXUAL VIOLENCE

Gender-based violence is a harmful act perpetrated against a person's will based on socially defined gender differences between males and females. Sexual and gender-based violence (SGBV) can occur outside a humanitarian or conflict setting. Conflict-related sexual violence (CRSV) refers to rape, sexual slavery, forced prostitution, forced pregnancy, forced abortion, enforced sterilisation, forced marriage, and any other form of sexual violence of comparable gravity perpetrated against women, men, girls, or boys that is directly or indirectly linked to a conflict. Whilst males may be affected by any of these forms of violence, violence is more often perpetrated against females. CRSV has been recognised by the UN as a peace and security issue that dramatically increases the social and societal harms from war and impedes the restoration of international peace and security. The UNSCR 2467 (2019) [19] mandates the UN

Secretary General to report annually on the implementation of UNSCRs 1820 (2008), 1888 (2009), 1960 (2010), and 2106 (2013). Civilian women and children may be the direct targets of state and non-state actors through the use of CRSV as an instrument of war. Women's voices are often excluded from the processes of peace-building and post-conflict political reconciliation. This has resulted in a concerted effort to increase the gender balance through the creation of the 'women in peace and security (WPS)' agenda. UN peacekeeping missions and many national armed forces have established WPS policies and developed training for 'women's protection advisers', CSRV specialists, and general personnel. There is also an acknowledgement that peacekeepers and humanitarian workers may themselves be perpetrators of forms of sexual violence. Please undertake Learning Activity 11.2 to review further resources and consider how the WPS agenda may contribute to reducing the violence against women and children during conflict and war. Chapter 13 will consider the provision of mental health services for victims of SGBV and CRSV in a humanitarian context.

Learning Activity 11.2   Case Study – Women, Peace, and Security?

The Women, Peace, and Security Agenda has been established to encourage full, equal, and meaningful participation of women in peace-making, conflict prevention, and peacebuilding efforts. Undertake a Google search using the phrase 'women peace security' and scan the sources of hits that cover policy, research, and analysis of the topic.

Read the most up-to-date annual report of the UN Special Representative of the Secretary-General on Sexual Violence in Conflict, available at `https://www.un.org/sexualviolenceinconflict/`

Scan the Handbook for United Nations Field Missions on Preventing and Responding to Conflict-Related Sexual Violence, available at `https://dppa.un.org/en/handbook-united-nations-field-missions-preventing-and-responding-to-conflict-related-sexual-violence`

Consider the following questions:

- What are the common elements of the recommendations of the annual report across all armed conflicts?
- What are the obligations of States to prevent and respond to CRSV?
- How might advisers in UN missions and national armed forces contribute to reducing CRSV?

LOOKING FORWARD

This chapter has provided an overview to the issues to be considered when providing health services for women and children in a humanitarian or conflict setting. There are many similarities between child and maternal health services and the 'chain of care' approach to trauma services. This emphasises the importance of a systems approach to organising health services and integrating services to meet the full range of needs of dependent populations. This chapter has also linked to Chapter 10, Communicable

Diseases, and has identified linkages with Chapter 13, Mental Health. The next chapter on non-communicable diseases (NCDs) will also highlight how many determinants of health and health behaviours that affect women and children will have an impact on the incidence of NCDs as they progress through their adult lives.

SOURCES AND RESOURCES

Suggested Internet search terms are as follows: 'sexual and reproductive health' or 'child health' and
'conflict' or 'war'.
Suggested websites and online sources for further information are as follows:
UN International Children's Emergency Fund (UNICEF). This is a UN agency responsible for providing humanitarian assistance and development aid to children in need. https://www.unicef.org/
World Health Organization

Pregnancy, Childbirth, Postpartum and Newborn Care: A guide for essential practice. https://www.who.int/publications/i/item/9789241549356

Managing complications in pregnancy and childbirth: A guide for midwives and doctors – Second Edition. https://www.who.int/publications/i/item/9789241565493

WHO Safe Childbirth Checklist. https://www.who.int/teams/integrated-health-services/patient-safety/research/safe-childbirth

Newborn Health in Humanitarian Settings Field Guide. Interagency Working Group on Reproductive Health in Crises. (2023) Available at https://newbornfieldguide.com/en/

Integrated management of childhood illness. https://www.who.int/teams/maternal-newborn-child-adolescent-health-and-ageing/child-health/integrated-management-of-childhood-illness

Vaccination in Humanitarian Emergencies. https://www.who.int/teams/immunization-vaccines-and-biologicals/essential-programme-on-immunization/implementation/vaccination-in-humanitarian-emergencies

Inter-Agency Working Group on Reproductive Health in Crises – https://iawg.net/ – this group aims to strengthen and expand access to quality SRH services for people affected by crises. It does this by evaluating the state of practice and producing guidelines and other material.

EQUAL – https://equalresearch.org/ – This is a multi-country research consortium generating evidence on effective approaches to deliver life-saving maternal and newborn healthcare in countries affected by conflict.

Alliance for Child Protection in Humanitarian Action – https://alliancecpha.org/ – a network of stakeholders for technical collaboration on child protection in humanitarian contexts.

Save the Children – `https://www.savethechildren.net/` – a global network of country-based fundraisers providing humanitarian response and development projects to meet the needs of children caught up in war zones and disasters.

War Child – `https://www.warchild.net/` – an advocacy network and services provider working to ensure no child is part of war.

Learning Activity 11.1   Incidence and Consequence of War on Women and Children – Suggested Answers

How do the video and the academic evidence of the impact of war on women and children make you feel?

Only you will know how this evidence makes you feel. You may reflect on the value of International Humanitarian Law and ethics that were discussed in Chapter 6 and how they might influence the decision-makers who control the behaviours of armed forces and non-state armed groups in their conduct of war and the use of violence. You might also reflect on what you learned from Chapter 7 and consider how the United Nations and its agencies and the wider humanitarian community work to prevent and mitigate the impact of war on women and children.

Learning Activity 11.2   Case Study – Women, Peace, and Security? Suggested Answers

Suggested answers are as follows:

- What are the common elements of the recommendations of annual report across all armed conflicts? Pages 17–44 of the 2024 report of the UN Secretary-General on CRSV (available at `https://www.un.org/sexualviolenceinconflict/wp-content/uploads/2024/05/SG-2023-annual-reportsmallFINAL.pdf`) cover CRSV in a range of conflict and humanitarian emergencies. The first recommendation for each country calls upon the governments and warring parties to implement the respective joint communique on CRSV, to respect human rights, and to undertake measures to reduce CRSV within their security forces and to investigate allegations of CRSV crimes.
- What are the obligations of states to prevent and respond to CRSV?

Pages 60–61 of the 2024 Annual Report on CRSV list the recommendations for Member States and wider stakeholders to reduce CRSV.

- How might advisers in UN missions and national armed forces contribute to reducing CRSV?
  The Handbook for United Nations Field Missions on Preventing and Responding to CRSV lists a large number of actions to be taken by UN missions to reduce CRSV. These include: advising and mainstreaming the topic; advocacy and capacity-building; monitoring, analysing and reporting; providing physical protection to prevent and respond; engagement with state and non-state parties to conflict; and ending impunity for perpetrators of CRSV.

NOTE

1. See pages 1–88 of the *Sphere Handbook*.

REFERENCES

1. Garry, S. and Checchi, F. (2020). Armed conflict and public health: into the 21st century. *Journal of Public Health* 42 (3): e287–e298. https://doi.org/10.1093/pubmed/fdz095.

2. Interagency Working Group on Reproductive Health in Crises (2023) Interagency field manual on reproductive health in humanitarian settings. https://iawgfieldmanual.com/manual and a summary guide to the MISP is available at: https://iawg.net/resources/misp-reference.

3. Vidler, M., Kinshella, M.W., Sevene, E. et al. (2023). Transitioning from the 'Three Delays' to a focus on continuity of care: a qualitative analysis of maternal deaths in rural Pakistan and Mozambique. *BMC Pregnancy Childbirth* 23 (1): 748. https://doi.org/10.1186/s12884-023-06055-w.

4. World Health Organization (2022). *Family Planning: A Global Handbook for Providers (2022 update)*. Department of Sexual and Reproductive Health and Research (WHO/SRH) and Johns Hopkins Bloomberg School of Public Health/Center for Communication Programs (CCP), Knowledge SUCCESS. Baltimore and Geneva: CCP and WHO https://fphandbook.org/sites/default/files/WHO–JHU–FPHandbook–2022Ed–v221115a.pdf and the FP Handbook website: https://fphandbook.org/.

5. Save the Children and UNFPA (2009). Adolescent sexual and reproductive health toolkit for humanitarian settings. https://www.unfpa.org/publications/adolescent–sexual–and–reproductive–health–toolkit–humanitarian–settings.

6. Singh, N.S., Ataullahjan, A., Ndiaye, K. et al. (2021). Delivering health interventions to women, children, and adolescents in conflict settings: what have we learned from ten country case studies? *The Lancet.* 397 (10273): 533–542. https://www.thelancet.com/journals/lancet/article/PIIS0140-6736(21)00132-X/fulltext.

7. IAWG (2023). Basic emergency obstetric and newborn care (BEmONC) in crisis settings. https://iawg.net/resources/basic-emergency-obstetric-and-newborn-care-bemonc-in-crisis-settings-select-signal-functions.

8. Medicins Sans Frontieres (2019). Essential obstetric and newborn care. Practical guide for midwives, doctors with obstetrics training and health care personnel who deal with obstetric emergencies. https://medicalguidelines.msf.org/en/node/449.

9. Interagency Working Group on Reproductive Health in Crises (2023). Newborn health in humanitarian settings field guide. https://newbornfieldguide.com/en/.

10. Rodo, M., Duclos, D., DeJong, J. et al. (2022). A systematic review of newborn health interventions in humanitarian settings. *BMJ Global Health.* 7 (7): e009082. https://doi.org/10.1136/bmjgh-2022-009082. PMID: 35777926; PMCID: PMC9252185.

11. Nguyen, D.T.N., Hughes, S., Egger, S. et al. (2019). Risk of childhood mortality associated with death of a mother in low-and-middle-income countries: a systematic review

and meta-analysis. *BMC Public Health.* 19 (1): 1281. https://doi.org/10.1186/s12889-019-7316-x. PMID: 31601205; PMCID: PMC6788023.

12. Martinez Garcia, D., Amsalu, R., Harkensee, C. et al. (2022). Humanitarian paediatrics: A statement of purpose. *PLOS Global Public Health.* 2 (12): e0001431. https://doi.org/10.1371/journal.pgph.0001431. PMID: 36962911; PMCID: PMC10021314.

13. Leach, K. and Checchi, F. (2022). The utilisation of vaccines in humanitarian crises, 2015–2019: a review of practice. *Vaccine.* 40 (21): 2970–2978. https://doi.org/10.1016/j.vaccine.2022.03.034.

14. WHO (2017). Vaccination in humanitarian emergencies. https://www.who.int/teams/immunization-vaccines-and-biologicals/essential-programme-on-immunization/implementation/vaccination-in-humanitarian-emergencies.

15. WHO (2008). Manual for the health care of children in humanitarian emergencies. https://www.who.int/publications/i/item/9789241596879.

16. WHO (2022). *Pocket Book of Primary Health Care for Children and Adolescents: Guidelines for Health Promotion, Disease Prevention and Management from the Newborn Period to Adolescence.* Copenhagen: WHO Regional Office for Europe https://www.who.int/europe/publications/i/item/9789289057622.

17. WHO (2013). *Pocket Book of Hospital Care for Children: Second Edition. Guidelines for the Management of Common Childhood Illnesses.* Geneva: WHO https://www.who.int/publications/i/item/978-92-4-154837-3#:~:text=It%20is%20for%20use%20by,of%20Childhood%20Illness%20(IMCI).

18. The Alliance for Child Protection in Humanitarian Action (2019). *Minimum Standards for Child Protection in Humanitarian Action*, 2019e. CPMS https://alliancecpha.org/en/CPMS_home.

19. United Nations (2019). S/RES/2467. https://www.un.org/shestandsforpeace/content/united-nations-security-council-resolution-2467-2019-sres24672019.

CHAPTER 12

War, Non-Communicable Disease, and Palliative Care

Richard Sullivan and Martin Bricknell

Centre for Conflict and Health Security, King's College London, London, UK

Abstract

The aim of this chapter is to review the provision of clinical services to care for non-communicable disease (NCD) patients and how to provide palliative care during war. NCDs cover hypertension, diabetes, renal failure, coronary vascular disease, chronic respiratory disease, and cancer. Although NCDs might be considered to be a hallmark of affluence, evidence from developed countries suggests that the adverse health effects of NCDs disproportionally affect people living in fragile and conflict-affected countries. NCDs are also long-term conditions that require continuing access to care and medication. When curative care is not possible, access to palliative care is essential to alleviate avoidable suffering. Continuity of care, supply of medicines, advanced diagnostics (e.g. CT and MRI scanners), capital-intensive therapies (e.g. radiotherapy), and availability of qualified personnel are all impacted by conflict. In addition, conflict-affected countries and post-conflict societies are often affected by the absence of regulatory frameworks, which balance commercial benefit with public health, leading to an influx of processed food products and a market opportunity for tobacco companies. Combined, these and other factors have serious consequences for NCD incidence and care. Patients in conflict settings have to navigate complex pathways of care using a mixture of public and private providers that may cross international boundaries. This complex network has been termed 'therapeutic geography' reflecting the lived experience of patients and healthcare workers living in conflict-impacted ecosystems. The topic of NCDs in conflict goes beyond humanitarian care, which focuses on basic primary care NCD medicines to include services that can only be delivered in hospital settings.

Handbook of Global Health, Security, and War, First Edition. Edited by Martin Bricknell and Richard Sullivan.
© 2025 John Wiley & Sons Ltd. Published 2025 by John Wiley & Sons Ltd.

Keywords: non-communicable disease, palliative care, social determinants of health, tobacco control

---

KEY LEARNING OUTCOMES

By studying this chapter, the reader will be able to:

- Define the wide variety of NCDs including their risk factors and how conflict mediates risk exposure, access and provision of care, and care itself
- Describe the wide variety of clinical interventions from primary care to hospital-based services needed for NCDs and how conflict ecosystems shape the access to these services as well as the capacity and capability of health-care systems to deliver them
- Specifically, describe how conflict shapes cancer care and palliative care
- Apply the concept of 'therapeutic geographies' through case examples of contemporary conflicts in the Middle East and Ukraine

---

INTRODUCTION

This chapter is based upon Section 2.6 Care of non-communicable diseases and Section 2.7 Palliative Care of the Health Chapter in the *Sphere Handbook* at pages 343–348. The key standards for non-communicable diseases and palliative care during a humanitarian emergency are as follows:

- People have access to preventive programmes, diagnostics, and essential therapies for acute complications and long-term management of non-communicable diseases.
- People have access to palliative and end-of-life care that relieves pain and suffering, maximises the comfort, dignity, and quality of life of patients, and provides support for family members.

NCDs represent an increasing burden of disease as the life expectancy of the global population increases. Whilst affluent countries have been developing preventive and curative health services to mitigate this increase, low- and middle-income countries (LMICs) have found it more difficult to regulate the industries (e.g. tobacco and food) which can have an adverse influence on health behaviours and more challenging to invest in preventive and curative services for NCDs. The populations affected by conflict and other humanitarian crises, now over two billion, reflect these wider influences with an increasing number of older civilians with chronic NCDs becoming displaced and losing access to care for long-term conditions. Please undertake Learning Activity 12.1 to understand why access to care for NCDs has become an increasingly prominent component of the health response to humanitarian crises.

Learning Activity 12.1   Why NCDs Are Important in Humanitarian Emergencies?

Watch: WHO/Noncommunicable diseases (NCDs) in humanitarian emergencies. At `https://www.youtube.com/watch?v=v-NQ0cLhko4`

Read: Bausch, F.J., Beran, D., Hering, H. et al. (2021). Operational considerations for the management of non-communicable diseases in humanitarian emergencies. *Conflict and Health* 15: 1–2. `https://doi.org/10.1186/s13031-021-00345-w`

Scan: Integrating Non-communicable Disease Care in Humanitarian Settings. UNHCR and IRC (2020). Available at: `https://www.unhcr.org/us/media/integrating-non-communicable-disease-care-humanitarian-settings-2020-pdf`

Consider the following questions:

- Which NCDs are most important in a humanitarian crisis and how do these patterns vary by situation and geography?
- How might the context of a humanitarian crisis exacerbate NCDs?
- What therapies and services should be included within a package of emergency care for NCDs across very different conflict ecosystems?

These questions are considered in the next sections of this chapter.

NON-COMMUNICABLE DISEASES

The priority NCDs in humanitarian settings are orientated around those that can be managed or mitigated through interventions in community and primary care settings through relatively simple medical and surgical interventions. The list commonly includes cardiovascular diseases (coronary heart disease, heart failure, and stroke), hypertension (raised blood pressure), asthma, chronic obstructive pulmonary disease (COPD), diabetes, and epilepsy. Renal disease is often excluded because of the challenges in providing access to renal dialysis. Cancer treatment is also excluded due to the technical challenges of delivering services that require complex diagnostics, surgery, radiotherapy, and/or a wide variety of cancer drugs, but it is important not to neglect the provision of palliative care (to be considered in the next section). Many of the determinants of health that influence the incidence of NCDs also influence the incidence of psychological and social ill health that will be covered in Chapter 13.

The majority of NCDs are mediated by the determinants of health as discussed in Chapter 1. The key environmental and behavioural determinants for NCDs are tobacco use, lack of physical activity, obesity causing foods, and alcohol and drug misuse. The impact of these determinants is mediated by socio-economic factors such as employment, housing, income, education, commercial marketing, and psycho-social stress. Conflict and humanitarian crisis settings can exacerbate the vulnerability of populations to adverse outcomes from NCDs due to the secondary impact on health systems or the tertiary impacts on the wider determinants of health. These factors may impact differently on different NCDs. An insulin-dependent (type 1) diabetic is at risk of serious complications or death if they are unable to access insulin for a few days, whereas a non-insulin-dependent (type 2) diabetic who has been well controlled on oral medication may not suffer significant complications if their drug supply is halted for a few weeks. The onset of health risks from a collapsed health system may also be relatively slow for cardiovascular disease and hypertension where the primary benefit of medication (e.g. anti-clotting drugs, cholesterol-lowering drugs, and drugs to lower blood pressure) is to reduce the risk of deterioration or a future acute event. However, the loss of hospital-based NCD services over a sustained period can have serious ramifications on the ability to manage new and pre-existing NCDs. As described by Roberts et al., the social determinants of health are also adversely affected by conflict or humanitarian crises, especially for displaced or refugee populations [1]. Tobacco (especially cigarettes), alcohol, and drug use can become a means of psychological and social solace. These commodities may become tradeable currencies if local money and international hard currencies become destabilised. The living environment may expose households to smoke from cooking fires and limit access to healthy foods and prevent appropriate physical exercise. Limited opportunities for work may restrict the purchasing power of communities, leading to exposure to dangerous and unhealthy workplaces, or even involvement in crime trading tobacco, alcohol, or drugs. Community and school-based health education may also be disrupted meaning that affected populations lose their health literacy and are unaware of options and choices for healthy living. Furthermore, these changes to the social determinants mean that patients are less likely to present early with new symptoms or a decompensation of a pre-existing NCD.

The WHO Package of Essential Noncommunicable (PEN) Disease Interventions for Primary Health Care provides guidance for health professionals working in primary care on the interventions for the major NCDs [2]. This has been augmented by the Package of Essential Non-Communicable Diseases Interventions for Humanitarian Settings (PEN-H) prepared on behalf of the International Rescue Committee [3]. Taken together, both documents provide a full review of each condition and recommendations for its management. These mirror arrangements for the management of NCDs in a peaceful and stable environment but balance recommendations for services with the realities of diversion of the health effort towards life-saving care for emergencies in trauma, communicable diseases, and maternal and child health.

PALLIATIVE CARE

Inevitably, the health response to conflict and humanitarian crises is focused on saving lives and mitigating the consequences of acute injuries and other medical conditions. However, communities affected by conflict and humanitarian crises may also include individuals with life-limiting acute or chronic diseases, including cancer. Curative treatment may not be possible for these people, but relief of suffering is an act of humanity which should be essential within the organisation and delivery of any type of health services.

Globally, cancer ranks as the second cause of death after cardiovascular disease both due to the increasing age of the population and longer lifetime exposures to cancer-causing agents (primarily smoking). Cancer is composed of three broad groups: solid adult cancers (bowel, breast, etc.), adult blood cancers, and childhood cancers. Many adult solid cancers, as well as other NCDs, can be prevented by a range of public health and preventative measures from immunisation against cancer-causing infections (e.g. hepatitis B and human papillomavirus), tobacco control, dietary interventions, through to population screening to detect asymptomatic early cancers (e.g. breast, bowel, and cervical cancer). For cancer to be cured, it has to be diagnosed and treated rapidly. This requires easy access to diagnosis and care as well as a wide range of diagnostic and therapeutic facilities. Different cancers require different combinations of the main modalities of treatment: surgery, radiotherapy, and chemotherapy. All these modalities, as well as pain relief medication (e.g. morphine), are also essential for palliative care. Cancer services are complex and expensive, requiring functional hospital-based services, or advanced clinic-based care facilities that are very vulnerable to disruption during conflict and humanitarian emergencies. Notably, some basic services, e.g. screening and treatment for cervical cancer and basic surgical cancer operations for early-stage bowel and breast cancers, can still be performed in humanitarian settings. Cancer patients from crisis-affected populations experience late presentation, delayed diagnosis, difficulty accessing treatment, and challenges with managing symptoms and receiving palliative care [4]. By some measures, cancer care can be considered to be a barometer for the functioning of a whole health system as these services are highly likely to be disrupted when priorities shift to acute health emergencies. Further work is underway to understand how better to integrate cancer into wider clinical services in conflict and humanitarian settings both in camps and within host country health services [5].

Palliative care covers the prevention and relief of the physical, psychological, social, or spiritual symptoms in patients and the support to their family [6]. The WHO Essential Package of Palliative Care for Humanitarian Emergencies and Crises (EP Hum) provides the reference point for the organisation of palliative care services [7]. This document particularly challenges the clinical approach to triage in emergency situations in which patients who will not survive given the availability of care (the expectant group) are given the lowest priority (see the discussion on triage in Chapter 8). It is suggested that this group should still be treated as a priority for the relief of suffering (palliative care) even if the goal of treatment is not to save their life. Thus, the principles of palliative care apply to all patients for whom the goal of treatment is the relief of symptoms rather than saving life or limb. This applies in trauma and other health emergencies (such as infectious disease outbreaks, e.g. Ebola or COVID-19) alongside the natural evolution of pre-existing terminal conditions. The relief of pain is the most fundamental component of palliative care. The allocation of supplies of pain-relieving drugs should be based on severity of pain rather than triage for life-saving treatment. There can be a particular problem in the provision of opioid-based pain medications (e.g. morphine) during crises because of the international regulatory requirements for their importation and distribution alongside internal national regulations around dispensing and record-keeping.

Palliative care for non-acute terminal conditions should be an integrated element within the holistic health services response to conflict and humanitarian emergencies. The EP Hum lists a range of inexpensive medicines that should be included within local formularies for the relief of terminal symptoms such as pain, shortness of breath, sickness, constipation, and mental distress. It also recommends that healthcare workers, mental health practitioners, and community social workers should be trained in the basics of palliative care covering all dimensions of health. It is particularly important to address anxiety and uncertainty around prognosis and disease progression through open communication to the patient and their carers.

THERAPEUTIC GEOGRAPHY

All of the chapters in this section of the book on health services take a public health approach to the ethical provision of health services on the basis of equity and justice in the allocation of resources to meet the needs of a population. These ethical principles were discussed in Chapter 6. These principles also have an implicit assumption that health services will be provided within the borders of a state. However, individual patients are often forced to seek access to health services on the basis of their personal assessment of need and their resources (e.g. political and financial), which can bypass the limitations of 'publicly' provided services. They may also cross international borders and seek healthcare in countries outside the area of crisis. Such cross-border healthcare may be facilitated or funded by UN organisations (e.g. the Exceptional Care Committees established by the United Nations High Commissioners for Refugees [8]), national overseas aid budgets, charities, or, most often, self-financed. This phenomenon has been called 'therapeutic geography' as a system-level explanation for patients' health-seeking behaviours [9]. It is distinct from medical tourism (in which individual patients are seeking healthcare on a commercial basis) and from refugee health (in which patients do not intend to return to their country of origin). It has particularly been observed for patients seeking treatment of war wounds and for cancer patients from Syria seeking access to clinical services in other countries within the geographic region (Lebanon, Jordan, or Iraq), though it has also been observed for patients from Afghanistan, Iraq, and Myanmar [10]. This has also been a feature of the European Union assistance programme to Ukraine where Ukrainian patients have been transferred to receive specialised care in hospitals across Europe [11]. The concept of therapeutic geography applies a patients' perspective to their access to healthcare recognising that there is a private/commercial market which may operate in parallel to the top-down government/humanitarian system. It is only through engaging with patients that it is possible to understand their personal experiences and choices associated with navigating complex health systems. This type of qualitative research makes it possible to interpret the lived realities of health-seeking populations affected by conflict and war.

RESTORING 'NORMAL' CLINICAL SERVICES

Chapter 1 discussed health systems in general and Chapter 8 described arrangements for inter-agency collaboration through the cluster system during the emergency phase of a humanitarian crisis. Chapter 2 introduced the concept of the 'Triple Nexus' in which humanitarian, development, and peace actors work together to co-ordinate activities during the post-conflict period as efforts shift from the external provision of humanitarian assistance towards co-production of strategies for rebuilding and development of health systems and services. Health services for NCDs, cancer care, and palliative care can be considered as part of the 'normal' provision of health services for a defined population. Thus, the foundations for these must be established or maintained during the emergency phase of humanitarian response so that they can be restored once the emergency demand for other types of health services (e.g. trauma and communicable disease) reduces to the pre-emergency baseline. Please undertake Learning Activity 12.2 to examine how the concepts from this chapter apply to access to cancer services for conflict-affected populations in the Middle East.

Learning Activity 12.2   Case Study – Restoring Cancer Services

Read the following papers about the characteristics of cancer services for conflict-affected populations in the Middle East.

Al-Ibraheem, A., Abdlkadir, A.S., Mohamedkhair, A. et al. (2022). Cancer diagnosis in areas of conflict. *Frontier in Oncology* 12: 1087476. https://doi.org/10.3389/fonc.2022.1087476. PMID: 36620568; PMCID: PMC9815758.

Akik, C., Asfahani, F., Elghossain, T. et al. (2022). Healthcare system responses to non-communicable diseases' needs of Syrian refugees: The cases of Jordan and Lebanon. *Journal of Migration and Health* 6: 100136. https://doi.org/10.1016/j.jmh.2022.100136. PMID: 36148323; PMCID: PMC9486618.

Skelton, M., Al-Mash'hadani, A.K., Abdul-Sater, Z. et al. (2023). War and oncology: cancer care in five Iraqi provinces impacted by the ISIL conflict. *Frontiers in Oncology* 13: 1151242. https://doi.org/10.3389/fonc.2023.1151242. PMID: 37213303; PMCID: PMC10196689.

Consider the following questions:

- What are the common impacts of conflict on local cancer services?
- What are the barriers to accessing care for local cancer patients?
- What are the routes by which cancer patients might seek care?

Suggested answers are at the end of the chapter.

LOOKING FORWARD

This chapter has provided an overview to the provision of health services for non-communicable diseases including cancer and palliative care. The 'physical health' chapters covering trauma, communicable disease, maternal and child health, and non-communicable diseases have shown how the delivery and recovery of clinical services after disruption due to conflict and other humanitarian emergencies is dependent on coherent strategies and policies across all stakeholders. This reinforces the importance of understanding health systems in general (Chapter 1) and how the health community might respond to crises (Chapter 8). This chapter has provided some insights into how the private/commercial sector can adapt and expand to meet the needs of patients if there is no public sector provision. This chapter has also shown how patients act as a 'market force' in their own right but are exposed to the risk of catastrophic financial costs in the event of a serious or complex illness. The restoration of a publicly provided package of essential health services aligned with the principles of universal health coverage is an important transition from emergency response to recovery and development. The next chapter will consider the mental health consequences of conflict and humanitarian emergencies and how health services should be designed to mitigate adverse outcomes in this dimension of health.

SOURCES AND RESOURCES

Suggested Internet search terms are as follows: 'non-communicable diseases' or 'cancer care' or 'palliative care' or 'therapeutic geography' or 'cross-border healthcare' and 'conflict' or 'humanitarian' or 'war'.

World Health Organization: Strengthening NCD integration in humanitarian emergencies. Available at `https://www.who.int/activities/strengthening-ncd-integration-in-humanitarian-emergencies`

NCD Alliance, available at `https://ncdalliance.org/` – this is a collaborative network that advocates and champions policy and practice in the prevention and treatment of NCDs.

PallCHASE, available at `https://pallchase.org/` – Palliative Care in Humanitarian Aid Situations and Emergencies. This is a network and partnership organisation that advocates for the integration of palliative care into the humanitarian response to emergencies by the development of standards, policies, and an evidence base.

A video of the practicalities of conducting a palliative needs assessment in a humanitarian setting is available at `https://www.youtube.com/watch?v=24uxyWseObk`

Learning Activity 12.1   Why NCDs Are Important in Humanitarian Emergencies?

Consider the following questions:

- Which NCDs are most important in a humanitarian crisis?
- How might the context of a humanitarian crisis exacerbate the risks from NCDs?
- What therapies should be included within a package of emergency care for NCDs?

These questions were considered in the sections 'Non-communicable Diseases' and 'Palliative Care' of this chapter.

Learning Activity 12.2   Case Study – Restoring Cancer Services – Suggested Answers

- What are the common impacts of conflict on local cancer services?
  - *Relative disinvestment in health in order to fund security*
  - *Diversion of health services towards trauma care and other emergency conditions rather than cancer*

(*continued*)

Learning Activity 12.2   Continued

- *Lack of personnel for cancer diagnosis and treatment – due to conscription, migration, collapse of training*
- *Destruction and lack of investment in diagnostic and treatment for cancer*
- *Sanctions and other regulations restricting the import and distribution of cancer drugs, medical equipment, and consumables*
- *Lack of technical personnel to support clinical services and maintain equipment*
- *Focus on private/commercial provision rather than publicly funded health services*
- *Prejudice against NCDs compared to support for maternal and child services*
- *Competition between NGOs and public sector services*
- What are the barriers to accessing care for local cancer patients?
  - *Awareness of symptoms and signs of cancer*
  - *Awareness of referral routes*
  - *Awareness of mechanisms for financial support*
  - *Safe travel to access services*
  - *Regulations and approvals for cross-border (internal and international) travel*
  - *Cost of travel and accommodation to reach services*
  - *Actual cost of services*
  - *Maintenance of personal medical records and follow-up*
- What are options for improving services?
  - *Development of insurance market to mitigate catastrophic financial hardship*
  - *Health education for awareness of symptoms/signs of early cancer*
  - *Training of cancer specialists*
  - *Investment in diagnostic and therapeutic capital equipment (possibly through private capital)*
  - *Financial incentives to draw health workers away from big cities/access to private practice*
  - *Creation of mobile electronic health records*
  - *Restoration/creation of cancer registries*
  - *Publication of standards, guidelines, procedures to increase consistency of services*
  - *Professional and financial support from diaspora and visiting experts*

REFERENCES

1. Roberts, B., Patel, P., and McKee, M. (2012). Noncommunicable diseases and post-conflict countries. *The Bulletin of the World Health Organization* 90 (1): 2–2A. https://doi.org/10.2471/BLT.11.098863. PMID: 22271954; PMCID: PMC3260582.
2. World Health Organization (2020). *WHO Package of Essential Noncommunicable (PEN) Disease Interventions for Primary Health Care.* Geneva: World Health Organization https://www.who.int/europe/publications/i/item/9789240009226.

3. IRC and USAID (2020). Package of Essential Non-Communicable Diseases Interventions for Humanitarian Settings (PEN-H). `https://www.rescue.org/report/package-essential-non-communicable-diseases-interventions-humanitarian-settings-pen-h`.

4. Shamieh, O., Kutluk, T., Fouad, F.M. et al. (2022). Editorial: Cancer care in areas of conflict. *Frontiers in Oncology* 12: 1087476. `https://doi.org/10.3389/fonc.2023.1301552`.

5. Ghebreyesus, T.A., Mired, D., Sullivan, R. et al. (2024). A manifesto on improving cancer care in conflict-impacted populations. *The Lancet* 404 (10451): 427. `https://doi.org/10.1016/s0140-6736(24)01023-7`.

6. Daubman, B.R., Khan, F., Slater, S.E., and Krakauer, E.L. (2023). Save lives and relieve suffering: the twin imperatives of humanitarian response and the role of palliative care. *Frontiers in Oncology* 13: 1120380. `https://doi.org/10.3389/fonc.2023.1120380`. PMID: 36937419; PMCID: PMC10019816.

7. World Health Organization (WHO) (2018). *Integrating Palliative Care & Symptom Relief into Responses to Humanitarian Emergencies & Crises: A WHO Guide*. Geneva: World Health Organization `https://apps.who.int/10665/274565/9789241514460-eng.pdf`.

8. UNHCR (2022). Guidelines for Referral Health Care in UNHCR Country Operations. `https://emergency.unhcr.org/sites/default/files/2024-01/guidelines-referral-health-care-unhcr-country-operations_1.pdf`.

9. Dewachi, O., Skelton, M., Nguyen, V.K. et al. (2014). Changing therapeutic geographies of the Iraqi and Syrian wars. *The Lancet*. 383 (9915): 449–457. `https://doi.org/10.1016/S0140-6736(13)62299`.

10. Baatz, R.K., Ekzayez, A., Meagher, K. et al. (2022). Cross-border strategies for access to healthcare in violent conflict – a scoping review. *Journal of Migration and Health* 5: 100093. `https://doi.org/10.1016/j.jmh.2022.100093`. PMID: 35373166; PMCID: PMC8971640.

11. Jackel, A. (2023). Combining efforts in medical support for Ukraine. European Military Medical Services. `https://military-medicine.com/article/4267-combining-efforts-in-medical-support-for-ukraine.html`.

CHAPTER 13

War and Mental Health

Rachael Gribble[1] and Martin Bricknell[2]

[1] Institute of Psychiatry, Psychology & Neuroscience, King's College London, London, UK

[2] Centre for Conflict and Health Security, King's College London, London, UK

Abstract

The aim of this chapter is to describe the impact of conflict and humanitarian crises on mental and social health and outline options for the provision of services for individuals and communities to improve outcomes. The chapter will outline the epidemiology, prevention, and treatment of mental ill health in conflict settings at individual and community levels. It will cover common psychological consequences of war and displacement, including post-traumatic stress disorder (PTSD), moral injury, and other mental health problems; the epidemiology of mental health problems in war-affected populations, including challenges in accurately assessing mental health; the societal health consequences of war and displacement and how this relates to mental health; mental health resilience; and treatment of mental health problems, including ensuring access to services through the provision of multi-layered services and identifying and overcoming barriers to accessing services. The case study will examine the realities of conducting research into mental and social health amongst conflict-affected communities such as Internally Displaced Persons (IDPs), refugees, and migrants.

Keywords: mental health, post-traumatic stress disorder, acute stress reaction, psychological resilience, moral injury

Handbook of Global Health, Security, and War, First Edition. Edited by Martin Bricknell and Richard Sullivan.

KEY LEARNING OUTCOMES

By studying this chapter, the reader will be able to:

- Describe the impacts of conflict on mental and social health among conflict-affected populations
- Understand the package of interventions within the phrase 'mental health and psychosocial support'
- Appraise the research evidence for the causes, impact, and interventions to treat and restore mental and social health of conflict-affected populations

---

INTRODUCTION

Chapter 1 introduced the WHO definition of health as a *'state of complete physical, mental and social well-being and not merely the absence of disease or infirmity'*. Chapter 4 highlighted the impact of population displacement on the mental health of internally displaced persons (IDPs), refugees, and migrants. The majority of Part 2 of this book is focused on physical health. However, mental ill health is considered in each of the 'physical health' chapters as a dimension of health need for these patients. Unfortunately, the term 'mental health' is most commonly used to refer to mental ill health, rather than positive dimensions of mental health. This chapter will use mental ill health to refer to mental health disorders but will also discuss resilience as a potential outcome of conflict-related trauma. In this context, the term trauma is derived from formal definitions of a traumatic event in the diagnosis of post-traumatic stress disorder (PTSD) in which an individual has been exposed to a serious/life-threatening physical event, physical or sexual assault or abuse, a serious health problem (e.g. intensive care admission or neonatal death), or torture. This exposure can be directly experienced, witnessed, or reported, as either an acute or repeated experience.

Conflict and humanitarian crises often involve multiple exposures to potentially traumatic events (PTEs). While PTSD and trauma are conceptually linked, trauma can give rise to other defined clinical conditions such as suicidal behaviours and self-harm, anxiety, depression, and substance (alcohol and drug) misuse. PTEs can also exacerbate major mental health conditions such as schizophrenia and bipolar disorder though it is not regarded as a directly causative factor. Mental health conditions can also be classified as mild, moderate, and severe depending on the impact on an individual's functioning within their social environment.

Whilst not a formal mental ill-health diagnosis, moral injury has emerged as a key concept within mental health and conflict [1]. It was introduced in Chapter 6 in the discussion on addressing ethical challenges during health crises. Moral injury refers to the psychological, social, cognitive, and spiritual impacts of perpetrating, witnessing or learning about events that transgress an individual's values and moral beliefs often as a result of perceived betrayal by a legitimate authority, hierarchy, or institution. Guilt, remorse, and shame feature heavily in moral injury. Moral injury is considered as a separate outcome from PTSD, but there is evidence to suggest that the two are linked and that moral injuries may help explain cases of PTSD that do not respond to usual forms of treatment. Much of the research on moral injury stems from research with military personnel and veterans in line with the work of Shay and Litz [2, 3]. Research continues into other high-risk occupations such as police, fire, and healthcare professionals [4] as well as an emerging body of literature relating to refugees and asylum-seekers [5].

This chapter is based upon Section 2.5 Mental Health of the Health Chapter in the *Sphere Handbook* at pages 339–343. The key standard for care of mental health during a humanitarian emergency is for people of all ages to have access to healthcare that addresses mental health conditions and associated impaired functioning. The actions are to:

- Coordinate mental health and psychosocial supports across sectors
- Develop programmes based on identified needs and resources, with consideration of vulnerable groups
- Work with community members, including marginalised people, to strengthen community self-help and social support
- Orient staff and volunteers on how to offer psychological first aid
- Make basic clinical mental healthcare available at every healthcare facility
- Make psychological interventions available where possible for people impaired by prolonged distress
- Protect the rights of people with severe mental health conditions in the community, hospitals, and institutions
- Minimise harm related to alcohol and drugs
- Take steps to develop a sustainable mental health system during early recovery planning and protracted crises

Please undertake Learning Activity 13.1 to reflect on the mental health consequences of war.

Learning Activity 13.1   Mental Health and War

Watch the YouTube Video: A life-saving intervention | Mental Health in Violence & War. ICRC at https://www.youtube.com/watch?v=MNvxrsWBWGA
Consider these questions:

- What groups does the International Committee of the Red Cross (ICRC) consider to be their target populations for Mental Health and Psychosocial Support (MHPSS) activities?
- What types of activities does the ICRC provide within an MHPSS programme?

Suggested answers are at the end of the chapter.

THE EPIDEMIOLOGY OF MENTAL ILL HEALTH DUE TO CONFLICT AND HUMANITARIAN CRISES: RESEARCH ON CIVILIANS AND MILITARY PERSONNEL

Despite the impact of exposure to conflict on mental health and the sheer number of civilians affected, the breadth and depth of academic literature in this area are far from complete. Much of the literature is based on refugees in high-income countries, excluding the experiences of the many millions more who seek sanctuary in countries nearest to their homeland or who remain displaced within their own country. Studies of refugees and asylum seekers often show high levels of poor mental health, including PTSD, as well as common mental disorders such as depression and anxiety. A recent study by Charlson et al., published in 2019, has estimated the prevalence of mental disorders (mild, moderate, or severe depression, anxiety, post-traumatic stress disorder, bipolar disorder, or schizophrenia) was 22.1% at any point in time for conflict-affected populations [6]. This estimate is broadly comparable to a meta-analysis of the prevalence of mental ill health in populations affected by fragility, conflict, and violence of 28.9% for depression, anxiety 30.7% and 23.5% for post-traumatic stress [7]. Alcohol and substance misuse may also emerge in some contexts, usually among men, as a means of managing and coping with stressors or poor mental health.

Many epidemiological surveys of the prevalence of mental health conditions use standardised questionnaires or interviews within populations in order to identify people with mental ill-health conditions. While these measures will capture Westernised conceptualisations of mental health like PTSD and depression, they may not capture other expressions of distress known as culturally related syndromes (CRSs) which may also be present within particular contexts. One such syndrome is *baksbat*, or 'broken courage', a psychological response to trauma experienced by Cambodian survivors of the Khmer Rouge, which includes facets of PTSD, anxiety, depression, and dissociative features [8]. Somatic symptoms, such as undiagnosable musculoskeletal or abdominal pain, fatigue, dizziness, and gastrointestinal symptoms, may also be more prominent symptoms of mental distress among non-Western populations.

The mental health consequences of conflict amongst members of the armed forces and their families have been the subject of extensive debate and a surge in academic study as a consequence of the effects of the NATO/US wars in Iraq and Afghanistan. This 'military' perspective has also influenced the understanding of the mental health consequences of conflict and humanitarian emergencies on affected civilian populations, from the conceptualisation of shell shock in World War I to the emergence of PTSD within DSM-III in 1980. More recently, this occupational approach has expanded to explore mental health among high-risk occupations such as police and firefighters, and healthcare and humanitarian workers who might be employed as part of an emergency response to a conflict or humanitarian crisis.

Mental health among uniformed services (armed forces and first responders) exposed to occupational traumas tends to be better compared to civilians exposed to similar events. This is because military personnel and high-risk occupations receive extensive training and, in many ways, have an inherent expectation that they will need to respond to dangerous and frightening events as a result of their work. These occupations also share a deep sense of bonding and belonging between workers, which allows for informal social support and understanding to be given within small groups such as a platoon or firegroup, as well as organisational support, which can involve early-stage interventions and clinical support as needed.

A recent paper by Petereit-Haack et al is one of many that summarises mental ill health in the armed forces and other trauma-exposed populations from an occupational health perspective [9]. This showed that soldiers deployed to war had double the risk of developing PTSD and 1.15 times the risk of developing depression compared to those without a war deployment. For US military personnel, it has been estimated that 14–16% of all personnel who deployed to Iraq or Afghanistan have developed PTSD or depression as a result [10]. UK research has also illustrated greater rates of PTSD among military personnel compared to the general population, especially those deployed on combat missions [11]. Petereit-Haack et al. also identified that rates of PTSD and common mental disorders are even higher among high-risk occupations, with workers exposed to occupational trauma three times more likely to develop PTSD and 1.73 times more likely to develop depression [12].

RISK FACTORS FOR CONFLICT-RELATED MENTAL ILL-HEALTH

The risk of an individual developing PTSD following trauma is a combination of pre-exposure, the trauma itself, and post-trauma factors. A narrative review of the literature on vulnerability factors of mental health in conflict-affected populations found that conflict-related violence and hardship itself have a causal effect on new mental health conditions, predominantly PTSD, depression, and anxiety. It can also exacerbate pre-existing mental health conditions. The segments of the population at most risk are those who are most marginalised: internally displaced people, children, women, the poor, elderly, disabled, and those with pre-existing mental health conditions [13]. Groups with particular experiences during conflict and violence such as torture, genocide, and sexual violence, and those with prior trauma, will also be more likely to develop mental health problems. Post-migration experiences can also adversely impact the mental health of refugee and asylum seekers, including issues with acceptance and integration, discrimination, difficulties with the asylum process, economic and working conditions, and a lack of social support and purpose [14].

Within populations exposed to conflict, more marginalised groups tend to be more at risk of developing poorer mental health due to greater exposure to violence or discrimination. These include women, children, and LGBT+ people. Chapter 11 on maternal and child health mentioned the specific mental challenges associated with caring for female victims of war. As a baseline, women tend to have poorer mental health than men, possibly due to socialisation, gender norms and roles, or gender-based violence. Although men and boys are also targeted during conflict, women and girls are also more likely to experience gender-based or sexual violence during war and civil disturbances, including rape, sexual assault, trafficking, forced pregnancy, forced marriage, and sexual humiliation. Such experiences may be specifically ordered by armed groups with rape used 'as a weapon of war'. Conflict-related sexual violence has extensive impacts on victims/survivors in terms of physical, mental, and social health [15].

Children are also vulnerable during conflict, as outlined in Chapter 11. A scoping, narrative review by Burgin et al. identified the additional mental health risks of exposure to conflict, humanitarian emergencies, and displacement compared to adults due to caregiver mental health, developmental impacts, and attachment issues [16]. Children may also be targeted by armed groups for forced participation in conflict as child 'soldiers' and both young girls and boys may be targeted for sexual violence. In addition to their personal experiences, the breakdown of social structures and education arising from conflict not only affects children's immediate mental health but can also affect their psychosocial development as they progress through childhood into adolescence and adulthood. Children forced into armed groups often experience a range of difficulties with reintegration on their release or return, with discrimination and stigma commonplace [17].

Children's expression of mental ill health is dependent on their age and social maturity. Among young children, it is highly unlikely that they can process, interpret, and describe their experiences and feelings in the same way as an adult. Indications of their distress may include social withdrawal, regressive behaviour, violence, prolonged crying, expression of morbid fears, and descriptions in art or writing. Older adolescents are likely to demonstrate symptoms similar to those of adults. The impact of exposures to trauma may affect their functioning as adults with consequential risk on the mental and social health to their adult interpersonal relationships and the mental and social health of their children.

Finally, members of the LGBT+ community may also be more at risk as a result of conflict. LGBT+ refugees can experience discrimination and verbal, physical, and sexual violence both before and during conflict from within their community and as they attempt to escape to safety [18]. LGBT+ civilians may be reticent to disclose their status when accessing healthcare, limiting their engagement with services, or engage in maladaptive coping strategies such as using drugs or alcohol and avoiding their cultural communities to prevent disclosure. Groups such as LGBT+ personnel may experience poorer mental health as a result of their minority status and particular experiences within military service [19].

Among military personnel and veterans, risk factors for PTSD also include aspects of marginalisation; younger age, race (non-Caucasian), education (low attainment), and lower military rank. It should be noted that some factors, such as male gender, may lead to elevated rates of mental ill health among infantry soldiers as this group is those with the most risk of exposure to trauma during deployments. Female personnel and those from the LGBT+ community may experience poorer mental health due to military sexual trauma and hazing.

Like civilians, PTSD severity among personnel and veterans is also linked to pre-military exposures (such as adverse childhood experiences, particularly physical or sexual abuse), the intensity of traumatic events, receiving a physical injury, or frequent exposure to traumatic events. Post-exposure factors such as unit leadership, inter-personal relationships, access to mental health services, stigma associated with mental ill-health, and post-exposure life events affect the risk of developing PTSD and its severity [20]. These risks are similar for other workers exposed to trauma (police, ambulance workers, war reporters).

THE IMPACT OF WAR ON SOCIAL HEALTH

War and armed conflict are hugely destructive to social groups and communities, often as a direct goal of the opposing force or group. Crucially, conflict reduces, limits, or prevents social support and social capital between individuals within communities. Social support is a key influence on health and well-being and one of the initial interventions attempted after any disaster. Through displacement, death, or injury, communities and the individuals within them can become detached, leading to poor mental health, reduced engagement with cultural practices, and an increase in anti-social and violent behaviours [21]. Specific groups may be targeted during ethnic cleansing and acts of genocide, leading to discrimination and stigma, preventing continuation of cultural beliefs and practices, and being subject to extreme violence or death. Gender-based violence may be used deliberately to play on cultural norms and values within targeted communities. Sexual violence not only causes mental and physical ill health as a result of the attack but can also lead to those affected being seen as 'contaminated' or 'weak', reducing their prospects for marriage and familyhood, further weakening community ties.

Research with Holocaust survivors has shown how trauma within one generation may impact subsequent generations through biological pathways of stress, alterations to gene expression, reduced cognition, and disrupted social roles or relationship templates [22]. Communities may also experience *collective* or *cultural trauma*, a social process through which trauma experienced at the group level (such as 9/11, the Holocaust, or Rwandan genocide), is reproduced and reconstructed in an attempt to make sense of it [23]. While collective/cultural trauma can give validity to the experiences of individuals and groups, and generate or lead to positive changes to collective identity, it can also perpetuate conflict and unrest where disagreements remain between perpetrators and victims.

CLINICALLY TREATING MENTAL ILL HEALTH DUE TO WAR

Mental ill-health and mental health services are often neglected compared to health services for physical conditions. In developed countries, intensive clinical interventions such as trauma-focused cognitive behaviour therapy (CBT) or other forms of trauma-responsive therapies show excellent efficacy for poor mental health arising from conflict [24]. However, in many LMICs and FCAS countries, mental ill-health services barely exist with very limited numbers of trained clinicians to meet the baseline demand. Not only may mental health needs in a conflict-exposed population exceed the capacity of mental health services, but pre-existing services may be reduced due to damage to infrastructure and migration or targeting of healthcare workers. Alternative interventions, such as narrative exposure therapy (NET), have been especially developed for use in refugee camps and under-resourced settings by lay practitioners and show excellent long-term effectiveness across a range of settings [25]. Civilians experiencing psychological distress may opt for treatment from traditional healers rather than clinical providers, especially where the disorder is culturally related.

The overall package of health services used in response to mental health conditions during conflict crises should be informed by the Inter-Agency Standing Committee (IASC) Reference Group Guidelines on Mental Health and Psychosocial Support in

Emergency Settings [26]. This describes a multi-sectoral, inter-agency framework for the effective coordination of organisations that provide MHPSS to communities affected by armed conflicts and natural disasters. These guidelines follow a similar pyramidal approach to interventions for all other health conditions with the foundation formed of basic services and security, and intervention layers of: family and community support; focused psychosocial support; general clinical services; and specialised services from psychologists, mental health nurses, and psychiatrists. Even more than for physical health conditions, MHPSS programmes emphasise the importance of non-health interventions from other response areas covered in the *Sphere Handbook* such as: protection (including social protection, legal protection, and codes of conduct); community mobilisation; food security and nutrition; shelter and settlement; and water and sanitation. These interventions stress the importance of community cultural, spiritual, and religious perspectives in the formulation, understanding, and approaches to treatment for mental health conditions, some of which may be very different from Western biomedical models. MHPSS interventions for children require even more cross-sector, multi-agency coordination than adult services, especially to use the education setting for community and peer interventions to enable resilience. Examples of holistic MPHSS programming for children are included in the UNICEF Global multisectoral operational framework for MHPSS of children, adolescents, and caregivers [27] and the Save the Children MHPSS Toolkit [28].

In parallel, the WHO mhGAP Humanitarian Intervention Guide (mhGAP-HIG) provides general guidance for non-specialist healthcare practitioners developed as part of the WHO Mental Health Gap Action Programme [29]. The mhGAP-HIG covers the particular context of acute and chronic emergency settings in which challenges such as limitations on time for training, access to specialist referral, and provision of drugs require the general mhGAP interventions to be adapted. The mhGAP-HIG is focussed on emergency clinical care for conflict-related mental ill-health conditions such as acute stress, PTSD, depression, and grief, and mental health emergencies such as suicide, psychosis, and epilepsy. The ICRC has published its own guidelines on MHPSS orientated to specific populations within a conflict context including families of missing persons, victims of violence, helpers, hospitalised wounded patients, detainees, and wider populations affected by emergencies [30]. There has been a substantial increase in the volume and quality of academic studies on the use of the mhGAP programme across global settings over the past decade [31].

RESILIENCE

Although an estimated 20–30% of people exposed to PTEs develop mental ill health, the majority of those do not. This suggests high levels of resilience, even among those exposed to multiple potentially traumatising events. However, it should be noted that resilience is not simply the absence of a mental health condition; many resilient people struggle with symptoms of poor mental health as a result of their experience and yet are also able to adapt to new environments and 'bounce back' or 'thrive' during exposure to additional trauma and adversity. While improvements to mental health are often the focus of interventions and clinical treatment, developing personal resilience should also be considered as a key outcome for those receiving support.

Post-traumatic growth (PTG) may be considered as a form of resilience that goes beyond merely a return to normal function and includes positive experiences developed from a trauma event [32]. PTG should not be considered as the opposite of PTSD as individuals may experience both, and instead, PTG encompasses meaning-making around the traumatic experiences people experience and how this may lead to the development of appreciation of life, more fulfilling relationships with others, new possibilities in life, greater personal strength, and spiritual change following trauma.

Finally, the concept of resilience can be relevant to communities and even nations in recovering from emergencies. Community resilience addresses the ability of a group, such as a town, village, or cultural group, to utilise available resources to respond to, withstand, and recover from adverse situations/stressors. This concept is situated largely within disaster research and climate change but may also be applicable in cases of conflict and war.

SPIRITUAL DIMENSIONS OF MENTAL ILL HEALTH DUE TO WAR

The cultural and spiritual determinants of health have significant implications for psychological health, and the framing of mental ill-health. Frameworks for MHPSS have explicit links to these dimensions as described in the IASC Guidelines on MHPSS and the *Sphere Handbook*. The spiritual or faith-sensitive dimension is a much more delicate topic because of the role of religious difference or intolerance as a contributing factor in the causes of conflicts. The term 'faith-sensitive' is often used to acknowledge the role of faith or religion within communities affected by conflict or humanitarian emergencies. It also recognises the contribution of faith or religion as a motivation for individuals or organisations within the network of humanitarian actors. A number of faith-based humanitarian organisations have published a faith-sensitive approach in humanitarian response for MHPSS programming to provide practical support for those who wish to be more sensitive to the faith perspectives and resources of the communities with whom they are working [33]. The role of faith groups in providing support to populations during the COVID-19 pandemic is an example of contribution that faith can have in the resilience of communities to crises [34]. Please undertake Learning Activity 13.2 to integrate many of the topics raised in this chapter by considering how you might help others in mental distress.

Learning Activity 13.2   Case Study – Psychological First Aid. How Can I Help?

Watch the IFRC video Psychological First Aid: Look Listen Link available at https://www.youtube.com/watch?v=c0YzDVIt9yg

Answer the following questions:

- What are the features of distress after trauma?
- How can you apply the 'look, listen, link' principles to yourself?

Suggested answers are at the end of the chapter.

LOOKING FORWARD

This chapter has provided an overview to the impact of war, conflict, and humanitarian emergencies on the mental health of affected populations, highlighting different mental health outcomes and discrete groups at greater risk of developing poorer mental health. The approach to the healthcare response to mental ill health is similar to the response for physical health conditions. However, the strategies and guidelines for MHPSS services place even stronger emphasis on the social (and spiritual) determinants of health by emphasising the importance of protection, security, community, shelter, food, water, work, and education in the mitigation of risks and consequence of war, conflict, and humanitarian emergencies on mental health. The next part of the book will consider how research informs the evidence presented as citations and references across this book and how evidence is used to advocate for policies at the organisational, national, and international levels.

SOURCES AND RESOURCES

Suggested Internet search terms are as follows: 'mental health', 'mental health and psychosocial support', 'MHPSS', 'child mental health', 'war', 'conflict', and 'humanitarian'.

Suggested websites and online sources for further information are as follows:
World Health Organization:

Mental Health. Available at `https://www.who.int/health-topics/mental-health#tab=tab_1`

Ensuring a coordinated and effective mental health response in emergencies. Available at: `https://www.who.int/activities/ensuring-a-coordinated-and-effective-mental-health-response-in-emergencies`

The Mental Health and Psychosocial Support Minimum Service Package. Available at `https://www.mhpssmsp.org/en-` website to support humanitarian actors to collaborate, plan, and implement MHPSS programmes.

IASC Reference Group on MHPSS in Emergency Settings. Website with multiple resources on MHPSS. Available at `https://interagencystandingcommittee.org/mental-health-and-psychosocial-support-emergency-settings`

The Mental Health & Psychosocial Support Network. Available at `https://www.mhpss.net/` – a platform for an online community of practice for MHPSS in challenging humanitarian and development contexts.

Beyond Conflict. Available at `https://beyond-conflict.co.uk/` – a UK-based network that advocates the need for mental health support for civilians in war zones and conflict scenarios and works to break down barriers to mental health access.

ARQ (previously the War Trauma Foundation). Available at `https://arq.org/en` – a Netherlands-based centre for prevention, treatment, and knowledge sharing on psychotrauma.

King's Centre for Military Health Research (KCMHR). Available at `https://kcmhr.org/` – the website of the leading military mental health research department in the United Kingdom.

Save the Children – What guides Save the Children's approach to MHPSS? Available at https://scintegratemhpss.com/approach/ – this is an online, multimedia summary of Save the Children's approach to providing MHPSS services.

War Child. Available at https://www.warchild.org.uk/ – War Child works exclusively to improve the resilience and well-being of children living with violence and armed conflict. Through their creative and evidence-based approach, they work exclusively to enhance the innate resilience of children and their communities.

Learning Activity 13.1   Mental Health and War – Suggested Answers

Consider these questions:

- What groups does the ICRC consider to be their target populations for MHPSS activities? *Victims of violence, people who have been wounded, helpers, families of missing persons, former detainees, and generally people affected by emergencies.*

- What types of activities does the ICRC provide within an MHPSS programme? *Social support, psychosocial support/psycho-education, mental health support (one-to-one and peer group), 'help the helpers' programme for first responders, counsellor for wounded children within a trauma-surgery support programme.*

Learning Activity 13.2   Case Study – Psychological First Aid. How Can I Help? Suggested Answers

Answer the following questions:

- What are the common features of distress after trauma? *Physical (e.g. shaking, sweating, and nausea), behavioural (e.g. isolation, crying, and eating changes), emotional (e.g. shock, fear, anger, and anxiety), cognitive (e.g. poor concentration, confusion, and forgetfulness).*

- How can *you apply the 'look, listen, link' principles to yourself? Recognise your own symptoms of distress, listen to yourself, link to self-care (e.g. peer support, exercise, and do things you enjoy).*

REFERENCES

1. Williamson, V., Stevelink, S.A.M., and Greenberg, N. (2018). Occupational moral injury and mental health: systematic review and meta-analysis. *The British Journal of Psychiatry* 212: 339–346. https://doi.org/10.1192/bjp.2018.55.

2. Shay, J. (2010). *Achilles in Vietnam: Combat Trauma and the Undoing of Character.* Simon & Schuster ISBN 978-0-684-81321-9.

3. Litz, B.T., Stein, N., Delaney, E. et al. (2009). Moral injury and moral repair in war veterans: a preliminary model and intervention strategy. *Clinical Psychology Review* 29 (8): 695–706. https://doi.org/10.1016/j.cpr.2009.07.003.

4. Williamson, V., Stevelink, S.A.M., and Greenberg, N. (2018). Occupational moral injury and mental health: systematic review and meta-analysis. *The British Journal of Psychiatry* 212: 339–346. https://doi.org/10.1192/bjp.2018.55.

5. Heide, F.J.J. and Olff, M. (2023). Widening the scope: defining and treating moral injury in diverse populations. *European Journal of Psychotraumatology* 2023 14: 2. https://doi.org/10.1080/20008066.2023.2196899.

6. Charlson, F., van Ommeren, M., Flaxman, A. et al. (2019). New WHO prevalence estimates of mental disorders in conflict settings: a systematic review and meta-analysis. *The Lancet.* 394 (10194): 240–248. https://doi.org/10.1016/S0140-6736(19)30934-1.

7. Lim, I.C.Z.Y., Tam, W.W.S., Chudzicka-Czupała, A. et al. (2022). Prevalence of depression, anxiety and post-traumatic stress in war- and conflict-afflicted areas: a meta-analysis. *Frontiers in Psychiatry* 13: 978703. https://doi.org/10.3389/fpsyt.2022.978703.

8. Chhim, S. (2013). *Baksbat* (broken courage): a trauma-based cultural syndrome in Cambodia. *Medical Anthropology* 32 (2): 160–173. https://doi.org/10.1080/01459740.2012.674078.

9. Petereit-Haack, G., Bolm-Audorff, U., Romero Starke, K., and Seidler, A. (2020). Occupational risk for post-traumatic stress disorder and trauma-related depression: a systematic review with meta-analysis. *International Journal of Environmental Research and Public Health* 17 (24): 9369. Available at: https://doi.org/10.3390/ijerph17249369.

10. Moore, M.J., Shawler, E., Jordan, C.H. et al. (2024). *Veteran and Military Mental Health Issues. [Updated 2023 Aug 17]. In: StatPearls [Internet].* Treasure Island, FL: StatPearls Publishing https://www.ncbi.nlm.nih.gov/books/NBK572092/.

11. Sharp, M.L., Franchini, S., Jones, M. et al. (2024) Health and Wellbeing Study of Serving and Ex-Serving UK Armed Forces Personnel: Phase 4 (2024). https://kcmhr.org/pdf/Phase_4_Health_and_Wellbeing_Cohort_Study_Report.pdf.

12. Petereit-Haack, G., Bolm-Audorff, U., Romero Starke, K., and Seidler, A. (2020). Occupational risk for post-traumatic stress disorder and trauma-related depression: a systematic review with meta-analysis. *International Journal of Environmental Research and Public Health* 17 (24): 9369. https://doi.org/10.3390/ijerph17249369.

13. Østergaard, M.L.D., Aponte-Canencio, D.M., Ortiz, Y.B. et al. (2023). Vulnerability factors in conflict-related mental health. *Medicine, Conflict, and Survival* 39 (1): 63–80. https://doi.org/10.1080/13623699.2022.2156232.

14. Jannesari, S., Hatch, S., Prina, M. et al. (2020). Post-migration social–environmental factors associated with mental health problems among asylum seekers: a systematic review. *Journal of Immigrant and Minority Health* 22: 1055–1064. https://doi.org/10.1007/s10903-020-01025-2.

15. Ba, I. and Bhopal, R.S. (2017). Physical, mental and social consequences in civilians who have experienced war-related sexual violence: a systematic review (1981–2014). *Public Health* 142: 121–135. https://doi.org/10.1016/j.puhe.2016.07.019. Epub 2016 Sep 10. PMID: 27622295.

16. Bürgin, D., Anagnostopoulos, D., Board and Policy Division of ESCAP et al. (2022). Impact of war and forced displacement on children's mental health-multilevel,

needs-oriented, and trauma-informed approaches. *European Child & Adolescent Psychiatry* 31 (6): 845–853. https://doi.org/10.1007/s00787-022-01974-z. PMID: 35286450; PMCID: PMC9209349.

17. Betancourt, T.S., Thomson, D.L., Brennan, R.T. et al. (2020). Stigma and acceptance of Sierra Leone's child soldiers: a prospective longitudinal study of adult mental health and social functioning. *Journal of the American Academy of Child and Adolescent Psychiatry* 59 (6): 715–726. https://doi.org/10.1016/j.jaac.2019.05.026. PMID: 31176749; PMCID: PMC6908764.

18. Nematy, A., Namer, Y., and Razum, O. (2023). LGBTQI + refugees' and asylum seekers' mental health: a qualitative systematic review. *Sexuality Research & Social Policy* 20: 636–663. https://doi.org/10.1007/s13178-022-00705-y.

19. Mark, K.M., McNamara, K.A., Gribble, R. et al. (2019). The health and well-being of LGBTQ serving and ex-serving personnel: a narrative review. *International Review of Psychiatry* 31 (1): 75–79. https://doi.org/10.1080/09540261.2019.1575190.

20. Forbes, D., Pedlar, D., Adler, A.B. et al. (2019). Treatment of military-related post-traumatic stress disorder: challenges, innovations, and the way forward. *International Review of Psychiatry* 31 (1): 95–110. https://doi.org/10.1080/09540261.2019.1595545.

21. Invisible Wounds (2017). Save the Children. https://reliefweb.int/report/syrian-arab-republic/invisible-wounds-impact-six-years-war-mental-health-syria-s-children.

22. Dashorst, P., Mooren, T.M., Kleber, R.J. et al. (2019). Intergenerational consequences of the Holocaust on offspring mental health: a systematic review of associated factors and mechanisms. *European Journal of Psychotraumatology* 10 (1): https://doi.org/10.1080/20008198.2019.1654065.

23. Hirschberger, G. (2018). Collective trauma and the social construction of meaning. *Frontiers in Psychology* 10 (9): 1441. https://doi.org/10.3389/fpsyg.2018.01441. PMID: 30147669; PMCID: PMC6095989.

24. Cognitive Behavioral Therapy (CBT) (2017). Clinical Practice Guideline. American Psychiatric Society. https://www.apa.org/ptsd-guideline/ptsd.pdf.

25. Siehl, S., Robjant, K., and Crombach, A. (2021). Systematic review and meta-analyses of the long-term efficacy of narrative exposure therapy for adults, children and perpetrators. *Psychotherapy Research* 31 (6): 695–710. https://doi.org/10.1080/10503307.2020.1847345. Epub 2020 Nov 18. PMID: 33205713.

26. Inter-Agency Standing Committee (IASC) (2007). IASC Guidelines on Mental Health and Psychosocial Support in Emergency Settings. Geneva: IASC. https://interagencystandingcommittee.org/iasc-task-force-mental-health-and-psychosocial-support-emergency-settings/iasc-guidelines-mental-health-and-psychosocial-support-emergency-settings-2007.

27. United Nations Children's Fund (2022). Global multisectoral operational framework for mental health and psychosocial support of children, adolescents and caregivers across settings. UNICEF, New York. https://www.unicef.org/reports/global-multisectoral-operational-framework.

28. Save the Children (2023). SCI Mental Health and Psychosocial Support Technical Guidance. London. `https://resourcecentre.savethechildren.net/document/sci-mental-health-and-psychosocial-support-technical-guidance/`.

29. World Health Organization and United Nations High Commissioner for Refugees (2015). mhGAP Humanitarian Intervention Guide (mhGAP-HIG): clinical management of mental, neurological and substance use conditions in humanitarian emergencies. V1.0 Geneva: WHO. `https://www.who.int/publications/i/item/9789241548922`.

30. ICRC (2020). Guidelines on mental health and psychosocial support. Geneva: ICRC. `https://www.icrc.org/en/publication/4311-guidelines-mental-health-and-psychosocial-support`.

31. Keynejad, R., Spagnolo, J., and Thornicroft, G. (2021). WHO mental health gap action programme (mhGAP) intervention guide: updated systematic review on evidence and impact. *Evidence-Based Mental Health* 24 (3): 124–130. `https://doi.org/10.1136/ebmental-2021-300254`. Epub ahead of print. PMID: 33903119; PMCID: PMC8311089.

32. Tedeschi, R.G. and Calhoun, L.G. (1995). *Trauma & Transformation: Growing in the Aftermath of Suffering.* Sage Publications, Inc. `https://doi.org/10.4135/9781483326931`.

33. The Lutheran World Federation and Islamic Relief Worldwide (2018). A faith-sensitive approach in humanitarian response: guidance on mental health and psychosocial programming. Geneva and Birmingham: LWF and IRW. `https://www.wvi.org/publications/development-guide/faith-and-development/faith-sensitive-approach-humanitarian-response`.

34. Goodwin, E. and Kraft, K. (2022). Mental health and spiritual well-being in humanitarian crises: the role of faith communities providing spiritual and psychosocial support during the COVID-19 pandemic. *The Journal of International Humanitarian Action* 7 (1): 21. `https://doi.org/10.1186/s41018-022-00127-w`. Epub 2022 Oct 18. PMID: 37519839; PMCID: PMC9579534.

PART 3

RESEARCH AND POLICY ADVOCACY FOR GLOBAL HEALTH, SECURITY, AND WAR

This third part discusses the opportunities and challenges of conducting research in the field of global health, security, and war in order to generate the evidence to inform policymaking at the national and global levels. Chapter 14 looks at the sources of research and other evidence of the impact of insecurity and war on the health of affected populations. The chapter reaches back to the chapters in Section 1 to consider how the evidence presented in those chapters was collected. It then considers the challenges associated with the conduct of clinical studies on patients in these circumstances. Chapter 15 examines the routes of influence that lead to policy formulation and how information is presented to political leaders and their policymakers in the process of policy formulation. It will also consider the limitations of the national and international systems in compelling compliance with a 'rules-based international system'. Chapter 16 concludes this book with some thoughts about the future of global health in the context of insecurity and war. Figure P3.1 is a picture commemorating the signing of the first Geneva Convention on 22 August 1864 in Geneva after a diplomatic conference hosted by Switzerland. Chapter 6 discussed the importance of the modern Geneva Conventions in setting international humanitarian law.

After completing this section, the reader will be able to

- Describe the opportunities and challenges associated with conducting research in global health, security, and war.

Handbook of Global Health, Security, and War, First Edition. Edited by Martin Bricknell and Richard Sullivan.
© 2025 John Wiley & Sons Ltd. Published 2025 by John Wiley & Sons Ltd.

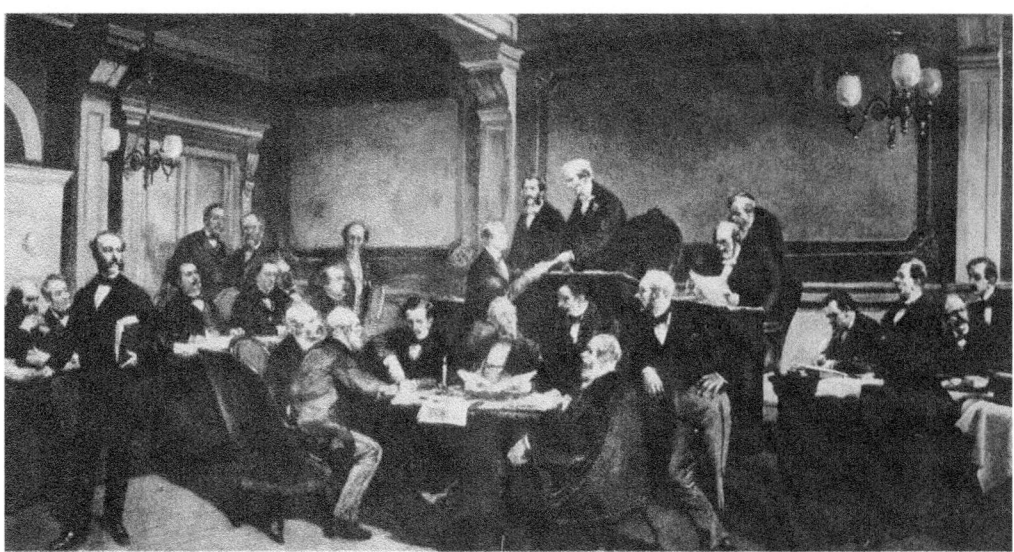

FIGURE P3.1 Signing of the first Geneva Convention. *Source*: Charles Édouard Armand-Dumaresq / https://commons.wikimedia.org/wiki/File:Signing_of_the_first_geneva_convention.jpg / last accessed February 07, 2025.

- Discuss the routes of influence that inform policy on the mitigation of the effects of insecurity and war on health.
- Summarise the inter-relationships between biomedical sciences and social sciences in the study of global health, insecurity, and war.
- Consider the evolution of this topic into the future.

CHAPTER 14

Research in Health and Security

Abdulkarim Ekzayez and Martin Bricknell

Centre for Conflict and Health Security, King's College London, London, UK

Abstract

The aim of this chapter is to examine the opportunities and challenges associated with conducting research in global health, security, and war. The chapter will open by considering how research and evidence have already been obtained and presented across the various chapters in this book. It will then summarise the key methods for collecting the data to generate this evidence and compare qualitative and quantitative methods. The next section will examine risks and threats to subjects and researchers in the context and environment of insecurity and war. The final part of this chapter will discuss how the findings from this research can be presented to inform policymakers.

Keywords: biomedical sciences, social sciences, literature review, quantitative research, qualitative research

---

KEY LEARNING OUTCOMES

By studying this chapter, the reader will be able to

- Describe the sources of evidence for the impact of war and insecurity on health

---

Handbook of Global Health, Security, and War, First Edition. Edited by Martin Bricknell and Richard Sullivan.
© 2025 John Wiley & Sons Ltd. Published 2025 by John Wiley & Sons Ltd.

- Examine how this evidence is created and the limitations on quality and quantity of data
- Identify the risks and threats to subjects and researchers in the conduct of such research
- Discuss how this research can be made accessible and presented to inform policymakers

INTRODUCTION

Knowledge can be defined as the condition of knowing about a topic through familiarity gained through experience or learning. This book has made extensive use of sources of evidence to illustrate the relationships between global health, security, and war in order for the reader to be equipped with knowledge. This evidence has been presented by citing academic papers, policy documents, commentaries, and opinion pieces. These documents use 'facts' in a variety of ways to support the arguments presented by the authors. This could be considered to be a process by which data (facts) are identified and collated. These processed data are then marshalled into coherent information that provides evidence for a particular perspective or conclusion.

Most chapters in Part 2 have opened by describing the number of cases of a medical condition (e.g. death, injuries, infections) within a defined group of people (population) associated with being exposed to the impact of insecurity and war. This approach uses **epidemiology** (the study of patterns of disease, derived from person, place, time in the investigation of diseases) and statistics to present information. Many chapters have then used policy documents or guidelines as a reference to a consensus amongst practitioners for the approaches to mitigate the impact of insecurity and war on affected populations through prevention, treatment, and recovery. In conflict-affected settings such as Syria, epidemiological methods have played a critical role in quantifying the health impacts of war and insecurity. For instance, during the polio outbreak in Syria between 2013 and 2016, surveillance data enabled the rapid identification of cases and guided the implementation of large-scale vaccination campaigns. These campaigns targeted children in hard-to-reach areas, leveraging local networks and cross-border coordination to ensure delivery under challenging circumstances [1, 2]. These real-world examples underscore the importance of using data-driven approaches to guide prevention, treatment, and recovery strategies amidst war and insecurity.

These types of guidelines represent a consensus amongst a group of experts on a topic. A guideline might include a summary of the academic literature on the topic as a formal '**literature review**'. Literature reviews have an academic method in their own right which includes a description of the process for identifying and selecting the literature to be reviewed and the approach to balancing the data and interpretation from each source. If the evidence relies on comparable statistics, it may be possible to combine the results of several papers into a '**meta-analysis**'. This approach is frequently used in biomedical sciences to compare therapeutic interventions (e.g. drugs or surgical operations) and the improvement on the health outcomes of study populations. If the evidence is not clear cut, or if there are a range of opinions on a topic, the process for gaining agreement may use a **consensus-building** technique that combines the knowledge of a range of experts. In addition to numeric information presented as statistics (**quantitative** information), evidence may be presented as narrative or opinion (**qualitative** information). Many research studies combine both approaches as '**mixed methods**'. Key concepts in research methods will be explained more fully in the section 'Key Concepts and Terms in Research'.

The Internet, search engines, and newly emerging artificial intelligence (AI) tools have transformed the access, management, and interpretation of information. This book has made extensive use of Internet searches and electronically archived material to develop the narrative and to increase the readers' access to information. A search engine uses computer algorithms to match the **search term** to the online information that is most likely to meet the user's request for information. In addition to Internet searches, it is also possible to search for information published in academic journals and books by searching bespoke academic databases such as Google Scholar, PubMed, Web of Science, and Scopus. Each academic database has a defined list of contributing academic journals and may focus on a particular academic field. Academic databases can search for article titles, keywords, author's names, author's affiliations, and other **meta-data**. Academic papers will reference their sources of information according to an agreed citation format (e.g. APA, Chicago, Vancouver). This enables a reader to find that source of information. Whilst electronic searching has transformed the access to academic literature, it is also subject to potential bias. Most academic literature has been published in English, in academic journals published in the Global North and on subjects relevant to this audience. This can result in a systemic bias that disenfranchises researchers and evidence from the Global South. Please undertake Learning Activity 14.1 as an opportunity to practice using search engines to find sources of evidence on conflict and health.

Learning Activity 14.1   Scanning Sources of Evidence in Health, Security, and War

Using the separate keyword pairs of 'health' AND 'security', 'health' AND 'conflict', and 'health' AND 'war', conduct a literature search for sources of evidence on the academic relationships between these keywords. Use Google (https://www.google.co.uk/), Google Scholar (https://scholar.google.com/), and PubMed (https://pubmed.ncbi.nlm.nih.gov/) (also consider Web of Science and Scopus if you have access). Compare the types of documents that have been identified in the first three pages of 'hits'.

Consider the following questions:

1. Is there a difference in the type of documents retrieved by each search engine?
2. What type of organisations publish documents in this field?
3. What type of academic journals publish papers in this field?
4. Are there any omissions in the coverage of the documents that can be identified?

Suggested answers are at the end of the chapter.

KEY CONCEPTS AND TERMS IN RESEARCH

This section will introduce key concepts and terms in the research of global health, security, and war. This topic straddles both biomedical sciences (including public health) and social sciences (including international relations, sociology, and psychology). This results in researchers having different philosophical perspectives and the research being published in a wide variety of academic journals. The research method can be categorised into two high-level groups: **quantitative** research, which applies statistical techniques to numerical data and is commonly used in medicine, economics, engineering; and **qualitative** research, which uses non-numerical data to understand individuals' attitudes, beliefs, or opinions and is commonly used in social sciences such as anthropology, sociology, and psychology and is often underpinned by sociological theories. Research can also be categorised as **empirical,** which uses observations, interviews, experiments to observe 'real life' and test or generate explanations of theories or concepts (e.g. reasons behind behavioural choices in smoking), or **experimental** in which the effects of an intervention are observed (e.g. a drug trial). Many of the papers cited in this book are **literature reviews** which summarise information from multiple academic papers or other sources to provide a summary of a topic.

Literature reviews can be divided into the following types:

Scoping review: A scoping review is a preliminary assessment of the nature and extent of research evidence on a topic which provides an overview and identifies knowledge gaps. These are often precursors to a systematic review [3].

Narrative review: A narrative review tends to be more comprehensive than a scoping review by providing a comprehensive synthesis of relevant literature to generate themes and topics. There may be some comparative discussion about the relative merits of individual academic papers though the analysis is primarily qualitative. These may not include grey literature and may have a risk of bias by being based on the opinions of single or a limited number of authors.

Systematic review: A systematic review will follow a proscribed structure using the Preferred Reporting Items for Systematic Reviews and Meta-Analysis (PRISMA) guidelines. These will have a specific objective, use defined search terms for identifying papers from online databases and explicit inclusion and exclusion criteria for inclusion of papers into the analysis. There will be a detailed comparative analysis of the papers, with an expectation of repeatability for the findings [4]. Where there are comparable data, this may be presented as a **meta-analysis** by pooling the data into a uniform statistical analysis. In principle, the findings of a systematic review are unbiased and repeatable by other researchers.

This book has made extensive use of common epidemiological terms used widely in public health.[1] These are defined below:

Incidence: The number of new cases within a population in a defined time period (e.g. the number of new diagnoses of COVID-19 by country per week).

Prevalence: The number of cases present within a population (e.g. the cumulative number of diagnoses of COVID-19 in a country at a certain date).

Absolute risk: The unique additional (or reduction) risk of a disease outcome from exposure to an external agent compared to a general population (e.g. the risk of dying from cancer in a lifetime compared to other causes of death)

Attributable risk: The disease rate in exposed persons minus that in unexposed persons (e.g. the incidence of dying from cancer due to smoking minus the overall incidence of death from cancer).

Relative risk: The ratio of the disease rate in exposed persons to that in people who are unexposed (e.g. the increase in risk of dying from cancer in smokers compared to non-smokers)

Epidemiological risks can indicate **causation**, a causal linkage between an exposure/intervention and an effect (e.g. smoking is a cause of cancer). Statistics can be used to test the likelihood of this linkage being true rather than due to a random association by chance. A theory of causation may be affected by **confounders**, the presence of a 'third' variable that has an independent impact on the observed effect. Examples are age, gender, occupation (e.g. older, male coal miners may have an independent risk of developing lung cancer compared to younger, female shop assistants independent of whether an individual from either group is a smoker). Many research projects try to exclude known confounders by matching characteristics between comparison study groups. Bradford Hill proposed a series of tests for causation beyond pure statistical analysis such as the strength of association, consistency of association between studies, specificity of the causable relationship (by time and dose response), and that the hypothesis is plausible, coherent with other knowledge, and proven by experiment [5].

The quality of epidemiological evidence will depend on the type of study. The most basic are **case reports or case series** where a researcher describes a new or unusual finding. This can then be tested using retrospective **case–control studies** (to determine relative risk) or **cohort studies** (to determine attributable risk). Where ethical, the hypothesis can be tested through prospective exposure studies that compare outcomes between control and observed (exposed) populations. The 'gold standard' for therapeutic intervention studies is the **double-blind randomised case control** (RCT) method in which the researchers do not know who has received the treatment and are not involved in the assessment of outcome.

Policy decisions are rarely made on the basis of a single research study. Indeed, the purpose of literature reviews is to identify and summarise multiple sources of evidence. The interpretation of such evidence into policy is often done using panels of experts to review and grade the evidence in support of their recommendations. The quality of evidence can be presented using a variety of hierarchies, and Table 14.1 shows an abridged example.

Within biomedical sciences, there has been a substantial effort to encourage researchers to improve the design and quality of reporting of research studies by standardising methods and establishing checklists for reviewers under the auspices of the Enhancing the Quality and Transparency of Health Research Network (EQUATOR Network). As examples, this group publishes the PRIMSA guidelines (cited earlier)

TABLE 14.1   Example of a hierarchy of research evidence.

Level	Type of evidence
1	Systematic review with meta-analysis of RCTs
2	Systematic review with comparability of cohort studies
3	Systematic review with comparability of case–control studies
4	Case series and/or poor quality cohort and case–control studies
5	Expert opinion based on first principles without empirical or experimental research evidence

and the Consolidated Standards of Reporting Trials (CONSORT) minimum set of recommendations for reporting results of randomised controlled trials [6]. Academic papers should follow the guidelines relevant to their type of paper.

READING A SOURCE OF EVIDENCE

The previous section summarised key concepts and terms in academic research. Analysing and interpreting evidence from a source of information is a core skill for an academic researcher. All forms of research and teaching require the state of knowledge on a particular topic to be summarised and critically reviewed. This section will describe an approach to assessing the quality and content of an academic paper. These principles can be applied to other information sources in both text and other media (e.g. video or audio).

Academic papers and grey literature are likely to conform to one of the following types of document: editorial, opinion/commentary, literature review, original research, advocacy proposal, policy brief, or implementation guidelines. Most academic journals will define the role of each of these types of papers in their guide to authors. Academic journals will also define their purpose, target audience, and relationship with academic societies or professional networks. The academic publishing market is highly dynamic and commercial with income based on either subscription (and access to papers controlled through payment firewalls) or open access with income derived from payments by authors for publication. Most journals operate a peer-review system by which each paper is reviewed by two or more academic peers who judge a submitted paper for quality and suitability for publication. The most prestigious journals have a high impact factor, and a low acceptance rate, are published in English, and are the target publication of the most reputable researchers in a field. Grey literature is more difficult to classify, though reliable sources provide a clear description of the publisher, their purpose, source of funding, and purpose of the publication. The critical analysis of an academic paper can be divided into four stages:

Stage 1: Review of the 'Meta-Data' – The first stage of critical analysis will determine whether the paper meets the researchers' 'inclusion' requirements. The algorithm of search engines ranks the listing results according to the likelihood of meeting the search string. In addition to the text of the search string, the search engine may also enable definition of the date range for publication and type of paper. The title and abstract in the listing will indicate whether the content is likely to meet the inclusion criteria. In determining the suitability of an individual paper, it is also important to consider: the journal (what is the ranking, scope, country of origin?), the authors (number, affiliations, contributor statement, reputation?), the source of funding (research agency, commercial, other?), the reporting of ethical approval (essential for human and experimental studies) and any conflict of interest statements. These factors will determine if the paper is likely to be of sufficient quality to merit full review.

Stage 2: Review of the Content – A biomedical sciences paper is likely to follow the 'classic' format of title, authors, abstract, introduction (which may include a 'background' section), methods, results, discussion, conclusions/recommendations, and references. The likely or expected content for each section is listed below:

Title: This should highlight the keywords/phrases relevant to the actual paper.

Abstract and Keywords: This is usually 300–500 words and should summarise the whole paper. The authors' choice of keywords may indicate how the topic of this paper links to the search string. Many journals specify a structured abstract for research papers.

Introduction: The introduction should explain the reason for the research, gaps in knowledge through a short summary of existing knowledge, and the specific aims and objective of the project. This should cite the key academic papers on this topic.

Method: This should explain the method chosen for the research including a description of the intended sample, the types of observations to be conducted, and the statistical or other approach to analysis of the results. This should cite at least one authoritative reference for the method and any research 'tools' to be used (laboratory assays, interview forms, validated surveys). It should be possible for another researcher to replicate the study based on the description of the method.

Results: This section will describe the findings from the research. It should include a summary of the demographics of the study sample, the data and analysis of the observations, and outcome of methods to exclude bias. The information may be presented as graphics or tables to aid the reader's understanding of the findings.

Discussion: This section will interpret the findings of this research within the context of pre-existing knowledge. It might be structured as key highlights, interpretation of main findings, strengths of this particular research study, and any weaknesses that limit the generalisability of the findings.

Conclusion/Recommendations: The conclusion may give an opinion as to the success of the project against the aims and objectives from the introduction. It could also make recommendations for further research or implementation of the findings into practice or policy.

References: The reference list should be sufficient and appropriate to the topic. Many journals limit the total number of references and so the list may not be comprehensive. The authors' previous work is likely to be cited but should not be excessive. Citations to non-peer-reviewed grey literature, new reports, and web pages should be treated with more caution than academic citations.

Stage 3: Triangulation with Existing Knowledge – The overall paper should be interpreted through triangulation with existing knowledge. A good quality paper will cover this in the discussion though it is likely to be favourably biased by the authors. It might be appropriate to check one or more of the citations to confirm the authors' interpretation. You should also reflect on whether the findings of the paper meet your intuitive understanding.

Stage 4: Critical Assessment – The final stage is your critical assessment of whether this paper adds to your own knowledge in the field and whether the findings are citable in the context of the purpose of your own search for information. This stage reflects the final step in the PRISMA process for the inclusion of a paper within a systematic review.

Please undertake Learning Activity 14.2 to critically analyse a literature review paper.

Learning Activity 14.2   Case Study – Critical Analysis of an Academic Literature Review

Using the four-step approach described above, review the following academic paper (previously cited in Chapter 11).

Baatz, R.K., Ekzayez, A., Meagher, K. et al. (2022). Cross-border strategies for access to healthcare in violent conflict – a scoping review. *Journal of Migration and Health* 5: 100093. https://doi.org/10.1016/j.jmh.2022.100093.

Suggested answers are at the end of the chapter.

CONDUCTING RESEARCH IN HEALTH AND SECURITY

It is important to increase the evidence and knowledge of the impact of insecurity and war on health, and the interventions that can mitigate these consequences through well-designed and implemented academic research. Unfortunately, such research is difficult because of lack of funding (relative to the scale of investment in research on the impact of conflict on the health of soldiers and veterans) and the practical challenges associated with safely conducting such research. It is vitally important that the approach to such research minimises the risk of harm to researchers and study populations (within the practical realities of operating in emergency environments) and is ethical. A review paper by Steinert et al. of the challenges associated with field research in LMICs highlighted a number of ethical challenges for researchers including clashes over roles, feelings of guilt, and emotional distress. This can result in actual mental ill health because researchers were emotionally drawn into the experiences of research subjects. These challenges were compounded by risks to physical safety, sexual harassment, and difficult working conditions [7]. The UNICEF and the UK Research and Innovation Council have recently (2021) co-published a guide for applicants for research funding on ethical research in conflict-affected countries [8]. These guidelines recognise that ethical considerations should be central to any research project but that these may be even more challenging in fragile and conflict-affected contexts. The structural power imbalances between local and international researchers can be increased, and the risk of harm to both researchers and study subjects can be magnified. The research setting may restrict the use of normal safeguards and the potential for coercive or unethical research can be increased. Although ethical approval is usually sought at the beginning of a research project, harm can occur throughout the research cycle even by excluding local collaborators from academic recognition in the final stages of writing up and dissemination for findings.

Researchers who work in fragile and conflict settings must recognise and mitigate any risks to their personal safety and accept that these risks may prevent or reduce the scope of their research. The researchers' host institution should have policies for risk assessment and management for researchers who work in challenging environments. An example of such a guideline was published by the Institute of Social Studies in 2016 [9]. This describes an approach to risk assessment covering security and health threats. These need to be mitigated by pre-travel preparations including security assessments using advice from national ministries of foreign affairs and travel health preparations (e.g. vaccinations and first aid training), and by obtaining and checking travel insurance including medical and emergency repatriation arrangements. During travel, the researcher needs to remain highly vigilant towards security and health risks including the risks of road accidents and hijack, the risks of robbery and assault, and the risks of contracting endemic diseases. On completion of the field research, the researcher must remain sensitive to the security of collaborators and research subjects (by being very cautious with personal information and contact details) and the presentational aspects of their findings (especially if this is critical of governments or institutions). They must also consider how they might access support for adverse impacts on their own physical or mental health.

Local researchers, particularly in contexts like Syria, often face heightened risks, including physical threats, coercion, and emotional distress, compared to international counterparts. For example, during the COVID-19 pandemic, local health researchers in northwest Syria conducted community-based surveys amidst aerial bombardments and with limited protective equipment [10]. Institutions must adopt equitable frameworks that provide tailored security training, mental health support, and fair authorship recognition for local collaborators. These measures ensure ethical and inclusive research practices, balancing risks with research outcomes.

DEVELOPING HEALTH AND SECURITY AS AN ACADEMIC TOPIC

This book has highlighted the global scale and distribution of populations affected by conflict and other humanitarian crises. The impact on human health from societal violence is catastrophic yet there is a lack of research funding and robust evidence to inform governments, international agencies, and NGOs on the best interventions to prevent and mitigate these consequences. Such research is difficult and dangerous to undertake but is an essential element of the global health effort. This research needs to be grounded in the needs, values, and resources of local communities. It should be undertaken in partnership with humanitarian actors and is an essential component of the monitoring and evaluation of humanitarian response, not an optional add-on. The journal BMC Conflict and Health published a collection 'Lessons from the field: Confronting the challenges of health research in humanitarian crises' in 2021.[4] The reader might consider reviewing this collection to consider what more needs to be done to promote academic research in the field of conflict and health.

This book and this chapter have shown how research in conflict and health crosses the professions of medicine, nursing, and health management. It also crosses academic disciplines in biomedical sciences and social sciences, employing research methodologies grounded in these fields. The best research programmes use mixed methods to capture the breadth of human experience while addressing the financial and practical barriers inherent in conflict settings. Innovative approaches, such as digital health tools, have been effectively employed in conflict settings to monitor disease outbreaks in real time despite limited infrastructure. Collaborative initiatives, like the Research for Health System Strengthening in Syria (R4HSSS) project, demonstrate the power of co-producing evidence by integrating local health directorates and international organisations. By prioritising context-sensitive approaches, these efforts provide a comprehensive understanding of health challenges and inform effective solutions. It is vital that such research adheres to the principles within the Humanitarian Charter in the Sphere Handbook, ensuring that research evidence promotes representation, engagement, and equity for the populations affected by these crises.

LOOKING FORWARD

This chapter has provided an overview to the creation of evidence through research in the topics of health, insecurity, and war. This augments the extensive use of research evidence to set the context for each of the preceding chapters. The next chapter will discuss how this evidence informs policy at national, regional, and global levels.

SOURCES AND RESOURCES

This chapter has already discussed how to approach the identification of sources and resources for research in health and security. Therefore, no further online resources have been added in this section.

Learning Activity 14.1   Scanning Sources of Evidence in Health, Security and War – Suggested Answers

Using the separate keyword pairs of 'health' and 'security', or 'health' and 'conflict', or 'health' and 'war', conduct a literature search for sources of evidence on the academic relationships between these keywords. Use Google (https://www.google.co.uk/), Google Scholar (https://scholar.google.com/) and

PubMed (`https://pubmed.ncbi.nlm.nih.gov/`) (also consider Web of Science and Scopus if you have access). Compare the types of documents that have been identified in the first three pages of 'hits'.

Suggested answers:

1. Is there a difference in the type of documents retrieved by each search engine?
   A Google™ search will find documents from all sources published on the internet. It will be skewed according to the location and language identified for the device that conducted the search. Google Scholar will identify documents published in academic journals and books. The default for this search is to sort by relevance, though it is also possible to sort by date. PubMed lists academic papers sourced from biomedical sciences journals.

2. What type of organisations publish documents in this field?
   - *Wikipedia*
   - *Government agencies including ministries of foreign affairs, ministries of health and development agencies*
   - *United Nations Agencies including WHO, UNHCR, and UNICEF*
   - *International organisations including the European Union, World Bank, and Pan-American Health Organisation*
   - *International NGOs including the ICRC, and International Rescue Committee*
   - *Think tanks, public networks, and consultancy organisation such as RAND, Chatham House, Global Health Information Network, Global Health Security Initiative, and International SOS*
   - *Academic institutions such as King's College London, Johns Hopkins, London School of Hygiene and Tropical Medicine, Liverpool School of Tropical Medicine*
   - *News outlets*

3. What type of academic journals publish papers in this field?
   - *Specialist journals: BMC Conflict and Health, Health Security, Lancet Global Health, Frontiers of Public Health, Military Medicine, BMJ Military Health, Global Health Action*
   - *Generalist journals: Lancet, British Medical Journal, Journal of the American Medical Association, PLOS one, Journal of Public Health, International Affairs*
   - *Books*

4. Are there any omissions in the coverage of the documents that have been identified?
   These searches only retrieve papers published in English; ideally, papers in Chinese, Spanish, French, and German would also be considered. The journals have to comply with formatting/access arrangements and so journals from non-'Western' sources may not be covered. Most authors are from the 'Global North', especially authors writing for think tanks and consultancies. There are often overlaps in 'literature reviews' published across the academic literature.

Learning Activity 14.2   Case Study – Critical Analysis of an Academic Paper – Suggested Answers

Using the four-step approach, review the following academic paper.

Baatz, R.K., Ekzayez, A., Meagher, K. et al. (2022). Cross-border strategies for access to healthcare in violent conflict – a scoping review. *Journal of Migration and Health*. 5: 100093. https://doi.org/10.1016/j.jmh.2022.100093.

Suggested answers.

Stage 1: Review of the 'Meta-Data'

Title: Describes the subject and type of paper

Authors: From three institutions including a specific research group

Abstract: Structured abstract, highlighting a formal research method

Journal: The Journal of Migration and Health is a broad-scope open-access journal publishing research, reviews, and other publication forms on any topics relevant to migration and health. It was first published in 2020 by the Elsevier publishing house as an electronic-only journal. The editorial board comes from a large number of international educational institutions. High likelihood of detection by academic search engines

Funding: Clear statement of source of funding. Open-access fees paid by research fund

Conflict of Interest: None declared

Cited by four other papers (indication of impact, number correct at the time of writing)

Stage 2: Review of the Content

Title: This highlights the keywords/phrases relevant to the paper – cross-border access to healthcare, scoping review

Abstract and Keywords: Structured abstract. Keywords that are linked to the themes in this book

Introduction: The introduction explains the reason for the research, noting populations affected by conflict may seek access to care outside the borders of a state. It also highlights the multiple potential healthcare providers. Identifies three research questions. Aim to propose a research agenda for further development of the concept. Provides key definitions for terms

Method: Explicit compliance with Joanna Briggs Institute Scoping Review Methodology. Includes 'academic literature' excludes other types of documents. Defines start year for search. Defines databases, search terms, and inclusion criteria

Results: Describes the process of down-selection to final group of papers. Defines the characteristics and categorisation for papers. Includes PRIMSA flow diagram in Figure 1. Narrative analysis of articles by research method and conceptual approach.

Discussion: Describes three themes arising from the papers, access to care, quality of care, and governance of care. Notes the limitations of the study – limited numbers of papers, omission of grey literature, only English language.

Conclusion/Recommendations: Proposes three principles and the themes for a research agenda. Notes the need for a better understanding of cross-border access to healthcare for conflict-affected populations and the need to improve the coverage and quality of future research.

References: Comprehensive set of references, though note the exclusion criteria.

Stage 3: Triangulation with Existing Knowledge

This paper has already been cited several times since publication. It is known that migrants and refugees may seek healthcare during their journey and in their new destination. The paper reinforces the reality that this healthcare is not solely provided by humanitarian relief organisation. The paper touches on concepts described in many chapters in this book.

Stage 4: Critical Assessment

This has the potential to be an important paper that could create a new agenda for the lived experience of populations displaced by violent conflict. It would be valuable to extend the research by including sources in other languages and from the grey literature.

NOTES

1. The UK Faculty of Public Health sponsors an excellence range of free resources in public health. https://www.healthknowledge.org.uk/.

2. Examples of high-status/high-impact biomedical sciences journals are as follows: *the New England Journal of Medicine, the Lancet, the Journal of the American Medical Association, Nature Medicine,* and *the British Medical Journal.*

3. An example is the country specific travel advice hosted by the UK Foreign, Commonwealth and Development Office. Available at https://www.gov.uk/foreign-travel-advice. The FCDO advises against travel to many FCAS countries and so researchers planning to go to these locations will require specific, specialist travel insurance.

4. Lessons from the field: Confronting the challenges of health research in humanitarian crises BMC Conflict and Health collection at https://www.biomedcentral.com/collections/lessonsfromthefield. The introduction to the collection is Mistry et al. [11].

REFERENCES

1. Tajaldin, B., Almilaji, K., Langton, P., and Sparrow, A. (2015). Defining polio: closing the gap in global surveillance. *Annals of Global Health* 81 (3): 386–395. https://doi.org/10.1016/j.aogh.2015.06.007.

2. Al Moujahed, A., Alahdab, F., Abolaban, H., and Beletsky, L. (2017). Polio in Syria: problem still not solved. *Avicenna Journal of Medicine* 07 (02): 64–66. https://doi.org/10.4103/AJM.AJM_173_16.

3. Tricco, A.C., Lillie, E., Zarin, W. et al. (2018). PRISMA extension for scoping reviews (PRISMA-ScR): checklist and explanation. *Annals of Internal medicine.* 169 (7): 467–473. https://doi.org/10.7326/M18-0850.

4. Page, M.J., McKenzie, J.E., Bossuyt, P.M. et al. (2020). The PRISMA statement: An updated guideline for reporting systematic reviews. *PLoS Medicine* 2021 (18): e1003583. https://doi.org/10.1371/journal.pmed.1003583.

5. Hill, A.B. (1965). The environment and disease: association or causation? *Proceedings of the Royal Society of Medicine* 58 (5): 295–300. PMID: 14283879; PMCID: PMC1898525.

6. Butcher, N.J., Monsour, A., Mew, E.J. et al. (2022). Guidelines for reporting outcomes in trial reports: the CONSORT-outcomes 2022 extension. *JAMA*. 328 (22): 2252–2264. https://doi.org/10.1001/jama.2022.21022.

7. Steinert, J.I., Nyarige, D.A., Jacobi, M. et al. (2021). A systematic review on ethical challenges of 'field' research in low-income and middle-income countries: respect, justice and beneficence for research staff? *BMJ Global Health* 6 (7): e005380. https://doi.org/10.1136/bmjgh-2021-005380.

8. Groves-Williams, L., Shanks, K. and Berman, G. (2021). Ethical research in fragile and conflict-affected contexts: guidelines for applicants. UNICEF and UKRI. https://www.ukri.org/wp-content/uploads/2021/11/UKRI-161121-Ethical-Research-in-Fragile-and-Conflict-Affected-Contexts-Guidelines-for-Applicants.pdf.

9. Hilhorst, D.J., Hodgson, L., Jansen, B., and Mena, R. (2016). Security guidelines for field researchers in complex, remote and hazardous places. International Institute of Social Studies. https://ihsa.info/security-guidelines-for-field-research-in-complex-remote-and-hazardous-places/.

10. Ekzayez, A., Al-Khalil, M., Jasiem, M. et al. (2020). COVID-19 response in northwest Syria: innovation and community engagement in a complex conflict. *Journal of Public Health* 42 (3): 504–509. https://doi.org/10.1093/pubmed/fdaa068.

11. Mistry, A.S., Kohrt, B.A., Beecroft, B. et al. (2021). Introduction to collection: confronting the challenges of health research in humanitarian crises. *Conflict and Health* 15: 38. https://doi.org/10.1186/s13031-021-00371-8.

CHAPTER 15

Policymaking in Health and Security

Ana Elisa Barbar and Martin Bricknell[1]

[1] Centre for Conflict and Health Security, King's College London, London, UK

Abstract

The aim of this chapter is to examine the routes of influence that inform policy on the mitigation of the effects of insecurity and war on health. This book has shown that the catastrophic effects of insecurity and war on health are well known. It has also shown that threats to health are a recognised risk within the range of threats to both global and national security. The mitigation of these threats has become an increasingly prominent element of health and security policy, especially after the COVID-19 crisis. This chapter will build upon the discussion in Chapter 2 about perspectives on security and consider how the evidence generated by researchers and practitioners in this field can influence the profile of health within security policymaking, and conversely, how considerations about war and insecurity must be included in health policymaking, even in peacetime. The chapter will open by considering how the impact of war and insecurity on health and health services is presented in the context of current wars. It will then look at how advocacy and influencing have placed this issue into national and global agendas. The final part will consider accountability, reaching back to the discussions on International Humanitarian Law (IHL) and ethics in Chapter 6.

Ana Elisa Barbar does not have an affiliation as she wrote this as an independent consultant.

Handbook of Global Health, Security, and War, First Edition. Edited by Martin Bricknell and Richard Sullivan.
© 2025 John Wiley & Sons Ltd. Published 2025 by John Wiley & Sons Ltd.

Keywords: health policy; policy formulation; political lobbying; war crimes

---

KEY LEARNING OUTCOMES

By studying this chapter, the reader will be able to:

- Describe the link between policy, strategy, process, and outcome
- Examine the role of evidence, the media, and messaging in the communication of the impact of war and insecurity on health and health services
- Identify the role of advocacy and the importance of influencing policymakers
- Discuss accountability within the global system to mitigate the impact of war and insecurity on health and health services

---

INTRODUCTION

At the time of writing this book, global international relations seemed to have become increasingly unstable. The full-scale war between Russia and Ukraine since 2022 has polarised relationships between Russia and the North Atlantic Treaty Organisation (NATO) Alliance. China has become progressively more assertive over its intention to unify Taiwan with the People's Republic and has raised tensions with other countries over the expansion of its maritime power. The Middle East is facing one of the region's longest periods of deep insecurity with the risk of drawing Iran into a sustained conflict in the region. The attack on Israel by Hamas in October 2023, the devastating armed offensive by Israel in the Gaza Strip and other Palestinian territories, tensions between Israel and Hezbollah on the border with Lebanon, and the fall of the autocratic Syrian regime have all created new levels of uncertainty in the Middle East. Africa is becoming more vulnerable to instability with a highly destructive civil war in Sudan and economic tensions threatening to cause popular unrest in many other countries. The civil war in Yemen and uprisings against the military government in Myanmar show no signs of diminishing. The consequences of these wars on affected populations continue to devastate families and communities. These examples show how war and insecurity change the security policy environment of countries and regions. Beyond the mobilisation of armed forces, martial law may be declared as a domestic policy, draconian restrictions may be applied to ethnic groups, and wider civil rights may be curtailed. Whatever the nature of security threats, governments and their agencies should comply with their national and international obligations in respect to human rights, international humanitarian law (IHL), and professional ethics (including healthcare).

Chapter 2 provided information and background reading on security theories and introduced some national security strategies. Chapter 7 discussed the term 'global health security', how health has become a topic within the security agenda, and how countries have refreshed their policies for mitigating catastrophic risks from health threats. Chapter 8 described health systems and how governments might have policies for emergency preparedness, resilience, response, and recovery for managing health emergencies. This chapter will examine the policy process in more detail and consider how evidence in the context of health, security, insecurity, and war influences policies and decisions by politicians and senior officials. These decisions affect the allocation of resources (money, people, time) to resolving security challenges by implementation of policies into strategies, processes, and procedures.

THE 'POLICY TO PRACTICE' PATHWAY

After the wars in Iraq and Afghanistan, the catastrophic West African Ebola crisis, and the management of the COVID-19 pandemic, some governments have started to reflect on their capacity to develop policies and strategies to achieve national objectives [1]. Policy development is an intrinsically human and political activity even if framed as a logical sequence of activities informed by evidence [2]. Stakeholders will try to influence the process through formal argument, often structured in written documents, alongside informal influencing. In government, policymakers may not be experts in their area of responsibility and will rely on subject matter experts to inform them and propose an agenda. Ultimately, policymaking involves choice, which is a political activity.

The 'strategy process' is often taught within national defence colleges and academies as a flow of analysis and decision-making, linking high-level policy to activity. This section will be based upon the 'Making Strategy Better' handbook from the United Kingdom Royal College of Defence Studies and uses a pathway to show how organisations may make decisions [3]. This model can be applied to test policies and strategies that cover health, security, and war. Figure 15.1 illustrates a 'policy to practice' pathway that shows how governments and other organisations create the organisational direction and activities to achieve their objectives.

Policy is a set of guiding principles, objectives or endpoints to be achieved in a domain of work, often reflecting the values of the policymakers, and forms the foundation for the development of strategy. **Strategy** is the selection of the approach, the assignment of ends (desired objectives), ways (routes to achieve the outcomes), and means (resources) to achieve the policy outcomes. Thus, a strategy can be considered as high-level plan that describes the framework to be applied to a problem and the allocation of resources (money, people, time). For security strategies, this is the allocation of the instruments of national power as described in Chapter 2. Strategies should be sufficiently longstanding and consistent that there is time for them to be disseminated, implemented, and performance observed before substantial change. This is often described as 'ends, ways, and means' to emphasise the importance of setting

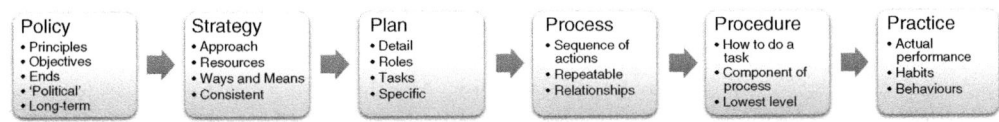

FIGURE 15.1   The policy to practice pathway.

clear policy objectives prior to starting the process of making strategy. A **plan** is a set of detailed instructions which inform individual elements of an organisation of their roles and tasks to contribute to the strategy. Implementing a plan will be dependent on business **processes** that describe the sequence and actions to be taken by organisations and teams to undertake a series of repeatable tasks. Ideally, the implementation of a plan will use established processes. A **procedure** is a detailed instruction for a task as an element of a process, and often applies to an individual or a small group of individuals. **Practice** is the actual approach to performing a procedure by individuals. Practice includes habits and behaviours alongside the detailed instructions within a procedure. Professions are grounded upon the practice to be expected by their members. Some authors have coined the adage: six Ps: prior planning prevents problems and poor performance.[1] Please undertake Learning Activity 15.1 to consider the difference between policy and strategy and how published documents influence the actions of stakeholders.

Learning Activity 15.1   Analysing Policy and Strategy

Using the suggested material or other documents of your choice, carry out the following tasks:

Policy documents: Find a government document on a health/security topic that is labelled as a 'policy'. Identify the problem that it addresses, the actions it directs, and the possible target audiences for this policy.

Suggested material:
Nigeria National Disaster Risk Management Policy [4]

Strategy documents: Find a government document of a health/security topic that is labelled as a 'strategy'. Identify the problem that it addresses, the actions it directs, and the possible target audiences for this strategy.

Suggested material:
U.S. Government Global Health Security Strategy 2024 [5]
In comparing these documents, is there a clear differentiation between policy and strategy?
Suggested answers are at the end of the chapter.

INFLUENCING POLICY

Policymaking is rarely undertaken by organisations in isolation. Chapter 2 discussed trends, threats and risks as the external context against which security policies are developed. This also applies to health policies. Whilst based on factual evidence, the interpretation and relative weighting of trends, threats, and risks is a qualitative judgement that frames the agenda for policymaking. Stakeholders might influence the negotiations of the agenda for a variety of reasons including economic or financial, socio-historical, political power, or moral beliefs. The subsequent selection of themes and structure for policy development is an inherently political (both interpersonal and philosophical) process that is constructed through complex engagements across a range of stakeholders. These may include politicians, advisers, civil servants, lobby groups, industries, financiers, pollsters, and public representatives. Their interests might vary or even contradict each other. Many national capitals host a network of foreign embassies, lobbyists, 'think tanks', consultancies, professional associations, and other groups, who seek to influence policies of government and inter-government organisations. Many models for policy and strategy development include a phase of 'stakeholder mapping' in order to determine the holders of political power and influence who should be engaged in the process. Consultation, in both public and closed sessions, is a critical element of policymaking and is often a legal or formal requirement.[2] The process of policymaking and the methods of influence are core elements of the study of political science, and the allocation and control of power in politics.

This book has cited multiple sources of policy within the text and has listed many additional sources and resources at the end of each chapter. Many of the non-government organisations listed, including humanitarian and peace-building organisations, have a significant advocacy or influencing component to their role which serves to maintain their political profile and to inform their access to grants and funding. Individual organisations may also operate as collaborative networks to increase their collective prominence, to share costs, and to build consensus in policy areas. Government organisations may also have advocacy or communication functions to facilitate acceptance of their policies and messages. The WHO has defined advocacy as

> a combination of social actions designed to gain political commitment, policy support, social acceptance and systems support for a particular goal or programme [6].

The World Federation of Public Health Associations (WFPHA) places advocacy as one of four enabling functions in the Global Charter for the Public's Health [7]. It is a key skill for practitioners of global health and public health as many determinants of health are influenced by politics, public policies, non-health services, and societal and individual behaviours. Advocacy techniques include establishing an evidence base, defining key or priority areas for the agenda, creating unified messages and products, establishing networks of stakeholders and supporters, developing media and communications channels, identifying opinion leaders and advocates, mobilising public support, and monitoring changes in the policy and operational environment.[3] This is much the same as any marketing or communications campaign. At the global level, a renewed interest in diplomacy for health topics has emerged since the COVID-19 pandemic and can be considered as the equivalent of state-based advocacy. It has been widely debated under the term 'health diplomacy', mobilising new efforts within the global health system towards more effective, sustainable, and concerted strategies in health, from the global arena to the regional and national initiatives [10].

CHALLENGES TO HEALTH POLICYMAKING IN THE FACE OF WAR AND INSECURITY

Many key national and global agreements, and policy conceptions have arisen through the influencing and advocacy of multiple stakeholders and organisations. Examples highlighted in this book include the Sustainable Development Goals, Universal Health Coverage, the Humanitarian Charter, the Sphere Handbook, and the Healthcare in Danger project. However, not all health advocacy is successful. The global progress on the SDGs is reversing, partly due to the impact of the COVID-19 pandemic on health outcomes but also due to the secondary economic impacts of the pandemic, the Russian war in Ukraine, and the impacts of climate change [11]. Not only are health goals affected by wider contextual circumstances, but the health benefits of public goods may be challenged by alternative vested interests. There have been criticisms of commercial industries for resisting legislation to control highly processed foods or tobacco products. The Ebola outbreaks of the last decade have demonstrated the importance of community mobilisation, collaboration, and engagement enabled by outreach and public communications [12]. The COVID-19 pandemic saw the public emergence of campaigns in social media and other outlets to discredit public policies including vaccinations. Legitimate alternative views may be amplified or distorted with the explicit intention to de-legitimise governments and public bodies [13].

The Internet and social media have created a supply of information that exceeds the capacity of governments, organisations, and individuals to analyse and process the information that they are receiving. This phenomenon has coined new terms such as infodemic,[4] misinformation, and disinformation.[5] Disinformation can be considered as the weaponisation of information and can be a tool used by adversaries during confrontation and conflict below the threshold of armed violence (see the Spectrum of Conflict in Chapter 2). There is an increasing recognition within public health that tools and procedures should be developed to help protect the authority and reputation of public bodies and to assist individuals to make choices beneficial to their own health [14]. A disinformation campaign could be considered as the reverse of an advocacy campaign. Please undertake the Case Study at Learning Activity 15.2 to consider the process of advocacy and lobbying for a new set of 'Pandemic Health Regulations'

Learning Activity 15.2   Case Study – Influencing a Pandemic Health Accord

The International Health Regulations (IHR) 2005 are designed to prevent, protect against, control, and provide a global health response to the international spread of disease in ways that balance public health risks against interference with international traffic and trade. The COVID-19 pandemic exposed weaknesses in the IHR and also opportunities for better global principles and co-ordination of a response to a pandemic. WHO Member States agreed to develop a Pandemic Accord, to prevent a repeat of the global health, economic, and social impacts of the COVID-19 pandemic through the establishment of an Intergovernmental Negotiating Body at a Special Session of the World Health Assembly in December 2021. The negotiating process during 2023 resulted in the submission of proposals to the 77th World Health Assembly in May 2024. It was agreed that the work should be completed by the 78th World Health Assembly in May 2025 [15].

Consider the following questions:

- Who are the stakeholders for a new Pandemic Accord?
- What are likely to be the limitations and risks of a new Pandemic Accord?
- What interests are at stake in these negotiations?
- How might advocacy and influencing work to support a new Pandemic Accord?

Suggested answers are at the end of the chapter.

In war and insecurity-affected contexts, bridging the security and health gap brings further challenges for policymakers. In insecure settings, the occurrence of human rights violations or political instability may hamper efforts to implement important health activities. In times of war, the government financial priorities might shift to security and military, reducing the focus, and the spending on public health interventions. Two recent examples demonstrate how the health response, from its policy and strategic aspects, was obliged to interact with security approaches. From January to November 2024, 33 countries had reported (or continued to report) cholera cases, with over 5,000 deaths due to the disease. Most of the affected countries are in conflict, or in a state of high insecurity due to violence. Yemen was the most affected country in 2024, and Haiti is the only country affected by the disease in the Americas region [16]. The global outbreak of monkey pox (mpox) has expanded from animal reservoirs in East, Central, and West Africa and was declared a Public Health Emergency of International Concern for a second time in August 2024. The Democratic Republic of Congo is one of the centres of transmission but has had the response to the outbreak constrained by the presence and uncooperative behaviour of armed groups, limited authority of government, and challenges for international organisations to negotiate between health and security actors to ensure an effective health response [17].

This book has emphasised the disruptive impact of attacks on healthcare on the health response and highlighted that these may amount to war crimes.[6] While several non-governmental organisations, certain states and the WHO have their own independent mechanisms to record attacks on healthcare to inform risk management, and operational decision-making and to increase accountability, there is a substantial debate on how such data capture should be done [18]. This policy debate is also a sensitive issue within the health and security arena, as it exposes the tensions between interests of states and those of the population affected by conflict or violence.

In closing, there can be clear gaps between health and security policies and implementation and accountability. Policies and strategies often miss these important components, leaving behind a gap on what, who, and how to approach these steps. Chapter 14 discussed how properly funded, formal research can assist in providing the evidence that shows the effectiveness, or not, of health and security policy.

LOOKING FORWARD

This chapter has provided an overview of the mitigation of the effects of insecurity and war on health through policies and strategies. It has considered the relationship between policy and strategy, and the indicative content of either or both. It has then looked at how policy is influenced by stakeholders through advocacy and lobbying. It has closed by considering opportunities and barriers to policy success, including the spread of misinformation and disinformation. The next chapter concludes this book by reflecting on the inter-relationships between biomedical sciences and social sciences in the study of global health, insecurity, and war, and considering the evolution of this topic into the future.

SOURCES AND RESOURCES

Suggested Internet search terms are as follows: 'advocacy' or 'lobbying' and 'global health' or 'global health security'.

This chapter has not provided any additional sources or resources because these are already provided in every other chapter of this book.

Learning Activity 15.1   Analysing Policy and Strategy – Suggested Answers

Using the suggested material or other documents of your choice, carry out the following tasks:

Policy documents: Find a government document on a health/security topic that is labelled as a 'policy'. Identify the problem that it addresses, the actions it directs, and the possible target audiences for this policy.

Suggested material:

Nigeria National Disaster Risk Management Policy

This policy document is aimed at national stakeholders from various governmental organisations, in the three levels of management. It may also be presenting the national coordination mechanisms to international stakeholders such as UN agencies, potential international donors and other states engaged in cooperation. The document describes Nigeria's comprehensive approach to disaster risk management and presents its position regarding coordination, and responsibilities of each response actor. It provides a framework for strengthening governance and implementation of an effective disaster risk response. In the health-security domain, this document presents some elements of vulnerabilities related to security (presence of conflict and armed groups, ethnic and religious extremism, etc.), and includes security actors in the disaster risk management process: military and security agencies are considered part of the response teams and have their responsibilities set out in the document. Also, security aspects are integrated as part of the management of the response, although without a clear definition of which activities should be considered.

Strategy documents: Find a government document of a health/security topic that is labelled as a 'strategy'. Identify the problem that it addresses, the actions it directs, and the possible target audiences for this strategy.

Suggested material:

U.S. Government Global Health Security Strategy 2024

This document was published by the White House and authored by the Bureau of Global Health Security and Diplomacy (GHSD) of the US Department of State (equivalent to a Ministry of Foreign Affairs). The Table of Contents follows the 'policy to practice' pathway. Chapter I described the vision (policy) and strategy statement. Chapter III sets out the approach/framework with three goals – strengthen global health security partnerships; catalyse political commitment, financing, and leadership; and increase linkage between health security and complementary programmes. The approaches/guiding principles can be considered to be policy statement. Chapters IV, V, and VI set out the plans and tasks for each of the goals. Annex 1 allocates tasks to individual government agencies, who will develop their own subordinate plans and processes. The annex includes a table for the allocation of money. This is an example of the integration of the elements of national power into a grand strategy for global health security.

In comparing these documents, is there a clear differentiation between policy and strategy? *In practice, there is a theoretical dispute between the primacy of policy or strategy. These documents fill both functions although they have different labels.*

Learning Activity 15.2   Case Study – Lobbying for a Pandemic Health Accord – Suggested Answers

The International Health Regulations (IHR) 2005 are designed to prevent, protect against, control and provide a global health response to the international spread of disease in ways that balance public health risks against interference with international traffic and trade. The COVID-19 pandemic exposed weaknesses in the IHR and also opportunities for better global principles and co-ordination of a response to a pandemic. WHO Member States agreed to develop a Pandemic Accord, to prevent a repeat of the global health, economic, and social impacts of the COVID-19 pandemic through the establishment of an Intergovernmental Negotiating Body at a Special Session of the World Health Assembly in December 2021. The negotiating process during 2023 resulted in the submission of proposals to the 77th World Health Assembly in May 2024. It was agreed that the work should be completed by the 78th World Health Assembly in May 2025 [15].

Consider the following questions:

- Who are the stakeholders for a new Pandemic Accord?
  This is intended to be a global accord signed by all members of the World Health Assembly. Thus, a list of stakeholders might include

(continued)

Learning Activity 15.2   Continued

Members of the World Health Assembly – national governments

The United Nations and subordinate agencies, especially the World Health Organization, each have a perspective.

Non-state actors in official relations with the WHO (219 organisations) – list of entities in official relations with WHO. Available at: https://www.who.int/publications/m/item/non-state-actors-in-official-relations-with-who

Economic and political alliances, such as the EU or ASEAN

Global organisations with an interest in health

National public health authorities

Biomedical sciences industries

Biomedical sciences academics

Informal, focussed consultations with experts – intergovernmental negotiating body/informal, focused consultations – https://inb.who.int/home/informal-focused-consultations

There were two public hearings in 2024 with an opportunity for a written component. Over 30,000 submissions were received. Intergovernmental negotiating body/public hearings – https://inb.who.int/home/public-hearings

- What are the challenges to be resolved in the development of a new Pandemic Accord?

Some examples:

Limits of the agreement – how much (or what is the minimal) substance should this agreement entail? Should it address all levels of work (prevention, preparedness, response, recovery) or focus on one of them?

Sovereignty – should WHO or other governments have the authority to override national sovereignty?

Accountability – who holds governments accountable for the implementation of the accord?

Compliance and oversight – how is compliance with the accords observed and measured?

Intellectual property rights – who owns pathogens, data, vaccine modalities? It includes a pathogen access and benefit-sharing (PABS) system.

Equity over sharing of resources – should the text include provision for a percentage of global stockpiles to be assigned to WHO? How would receiving parties be prioritised? Who would distribute the goods?

Financing – should the text include provisions for financing, including capacity-building for surveillance and laboratory analysis in LMICs?

Bringing 'One Health' into the accord – will plant and animal health threats be included alongside human health?

Timeliness – how to manage the risk of watering down provisions as memories of the COVID-19 pandemic fade? How to ensure the agreement is sufficiently debated, without dragging its approval?

- How might advocacy and influencing work to support or undermine a new Pandemic Accord?
There is a wide range of possibilities for advocacy and influencing to support such an accord. Please see some ideas below:

Support:

- *Promote the key features and value of the new Pandemic Accord to protect health and provide global equity in the response to a new pandemic*
- *Ensure key aspects of the agenda are not forgotten by negotiators*
- *Ensure technical aspects of the agenda are translated properly into the agreement*
- *Ensure technical, political and operational information is available to those who will need to frame and negotiate the text*
- *Ensure there is active balancing of political and financial pressures against social and welfare interests*
- *Reduce or mitigate disinformation*
- *Enable participation of minority groups or socially marginalised populations in the debate, such as autochthone populations, displaced persons or refugees, people living with disabilities, etc.*

Challenge:

- *Disinformation (disinformation has already impacted the ideals within the original proposals with some countries/organisations wanting to minimise the authority of the WHO to act on behalf of the global community over the sovereignty of governments [19].)*
- *Direct lobbying by stakeholders with heavy political or financial interests, yet disrespecting human rights*
- *Polarisation of the agenda with opposing arguments and lack of flexibility to dialogue*
- *Securitisation of response to a pandemic in place of a public good*
- *Already-used text formulas that result in empty or ineffective implementation*
- *Withdrawal of the United States from the World Health Organization*

NOTES

1. Readers may also know of another version of the adage: 'prior planning prevents pxxxxx poor performance'.
2. An example of consultation is the 2024 call for evidence for the Strategic Defence Review by the UK government. Available at https://www.gov.uk/government/calls-for-evidence/strategic-defence-review-2024-call-for-evidence.
3. Examples of approaches to advocacy include Refs. [8, 9].

4. The WHO defines an infodemic is too much information including false or misleading information in digital and physical environments during a disease outbreak. Available at https://www.who.int/health-topics/infodemic#tab=tab_1.

5. Misinformation is the spread of false information without the intent to mislead. Those who share the misinformation may believe it is true, useful or interesting, and have no malicious intent towards the recipients they are sharing it with. Disinformation is designed or spread with full knowledge of it being false (information has been manipulated), as part of an intention to deceive and cause harm. The motivations can be economic gain, ideological, religious, political or in support of a social agenda among others. Both misinformation and disinformation may cause harm, which comprises threats to decision-making processes as well as health, environment or security. Available at https://www.who.int/news-room/questions-and-answers/item/disinformation-and-public-health.

6. To learn more about what are attacks on healthcare, please access WHO's Q&A: https://www.who.int/news-room/questions-and-answers/item/attacks-on-health-care-initiative.

REFERENCES

1. The Stationary Office (2010). Who does UK National Strategy? House of Commons Public Administration Select Committee HC435. London: The Stationary Office. 12 October 2010. https://publications.parliament.uk/pa/cm201011/cmselect/cmpubadm/435/43502.htm.

2. de Leeuw, E., Clavier, C., and Breton, E. (2014). Health policy – why research it and how: health political science. *Health Research Policy and Systems* **12**: 55. https://doi.org/10.1186/1478-4505-12-55.

3. Defence Academy of the United Kingdom (2023). Making strategy better. Royal College of Defence Studies. Shrivenham: Defence Academy of the United Kingdom. https://www.da.mod.uk/__data/assets/pdf_file/0029/119594/2023_RCDS_STRAT_HDB-V15.pdf.

4. National Emergency Management Agency (2018). Nigeria disaster risk management policy. https://nema.gov.ng/documentations/National%20Disaster%20Risk%20Management%20Policy.pdf.

5. U.S. Government Global Health Security Strategy (2024). United States Global Health Security Partnerships. Washington, DC: White House. https://www.state.gov/united-states-global-health-security-partnerships/.

6. World Health Organization 1992. Advocacy strategies for health and development: development communication in action. Geneva: World Health Organization. https://iris.who.int/handle/10665/70051.

7. Lomazzi, M. (2016). A Global Charter for the Public's Health—the public health system: role, functions, competencies and education requirements. *The European Journal of Public Health*. 26 (2): 210–212. https://doi.org/10.1093/eurpub/ckw011.

8. Global Health Advocacy Incubator (2023). Advocacy action guide four phases to health policy success. https://www.advocacyincubator.org/resources/advocacy-tools.

9. Stoneham, M., Vidler, A., and Edmunds, M. (2019). *Advocacy in Action: A Toolkit for Public Health Professionals*, 4e. Public Health Advocacy Institute of Western Australia https://www.phaiwa.org.au/wp-content/uploads/2019/09/2019_Advocacy-in-Action-A-Toolkit-for-Public-Health-Professionals-1.pdf.

10. Falqui, L., Li, F., and Xue, Y. (2024). Global health diplomacy in humanitarian action. *Conflict and Health* 18: 46. https://doi.org/10.1186/s13031-024-00605-5.

11. United Nations (2024). The sustainable development goals report. New York: United Nations. https://unstats.un.org/sdgs/report/2024/.

12. Cénat, J.M., Broussard, C., Darius, W.P. et al. (2023). Social mobilization, education, and prevention of the Ebola virus disease: a scoping review. *Preventive Medicine* 166: 107328. https://doi.org/10.1016/j.ypmed.2022.107328.

13. Kisa, S. and Kisa, A. (2024). A comprehensive analysis of COVID-19 misinformation, public health impacts, and communication strategies: scoping review. *Journal of Medical Internet Research* 26: e56931. https://www.jmir.org/2024/1/e56931. https://doi.org/10.2196/56931.

14. Ishizumi, A., Kolis, J., Abad, N. et al. (2024). Beyond misinformation: developing a public health prevention framework for managing information ecosystems. *The Lancet Public Health.* 9 (6): e397–e406. https://doi.org/10.1016/S2468-2667(24)00031-8.

15. WHO. Intergovernmental negotiating body. Geneva: WHO. https://inb.who.int/.

16. World Health Organization (2024). Multi-country outbreak of cholera, external situation report n. 21. https://reliefweb.int/report/democratic-republic-congo/multi-country-outbreak-cholera-external-situation-report-21-published-18-december-2024#:~:text=From%201%20January%20to%2024,the%20same%20month%20in%20 2023.

17. United Nations (2024). DR Congo: conflict escalation linked to deadly Mpox threat. Press release. Geneva: United Nations. July 2024. https://news.un.org/en/story/2024/07/1152031.

18. International Peace Institute (2022). Strengthening data to protect healthcare in conflict zones. New York: IPI. https://www.ipinst.org/wp-content/uploads/2022/11/1120_Strengthening-Data-on-Attacks-on-Healthcare.pdf.

19. Soliman, A., Taguchi, K., Matsoso, P. et al. (2023). WHO pandemic accord: full adherence to the principle of sovereignty. *The Lancet.* 402 (10410): 1322–1323. https://doi.org/10.1016/S0140-6736(23)02018-4.

CHAPTER 16

Conclusions and Looking Forward

Richard Sullivan and Martin Bricknell

Centre for Conflict and Health Security, King's College London, London, UK

Abstract

The aim of this chapter is to reflect on the inter-relationships between biomedical sciences and social sciences in the study of global health, security, and war and to consider the evolution of this topic into the future. The chapter will use the lenses of health and security presented in this book to consider the global experience of the COVID-19 pandemic, the war in Ukraine, and the war between Israel and Hamas in Gaza. The chapter will next consider whether the contemporary experience of affected populations reflects the enduring nature of human suffering associated with insecurity and war or whether the current character of the instruments of political conflict is increasing the inhumanity of these consequences. It will close by considering the employment and career opportunities in this field.

Keywords: global health, health threats, COVID-19 security, Ukraine war, Gaza war, nature of war, character of war

Handbook of Global Health, Security, and War, First Edition. Edited by Martin Bricknell and Richard Sullivan.
© 2025 John Wiley & Sons Ltd. Published 2025 by John Wiley & Sons Ltd.

KEY LEARNING OUTCOMES

By studying this chapter, the reader will be able to:

- Interpret three contemporary security crises, the COVID-19 pandemic, the war in Ukraine, and the recent war in the Middle East through the lenses of health and security
- Examine whether the impacts of war and insecurity on health and health services reflect the enduring nature of political conflict or whether the character of these conflicts is increasing the inhumanity of war
- Consider how to seek employment in this field

INTRODUCTION

This book intended to engage the reader with multiple perspectives of the relationships between security and health. It was set from a global perspective, whilst acknowledging the referent perspectives of national security and human security. Thus, this book covered much more than the narrow definition of 'global health security' (GHS) as a public health response to threats from infectious diseases. It also examined the health consequences of the ultimate form of insecurity, war. Figure 16.1 was included in the introduction of this book to provide a visualisation of these different perspectives on the topics of health and security.

Part 1 presented different perspectives on health and security. It drew on key concepts from the fields of global health, public health, international relations, security studies, international humanitarian law, healthcare ethics, and military ethics. Whilst not authoritative on any of these fields, the section provided access to these perspectives from each individual discipline so as to strengthen an interdisciplinary understanding. Part 2 examined the impact of conflict and other health emergencies on different clinical services within a health system. The topics selected are those from the chapter on Health within

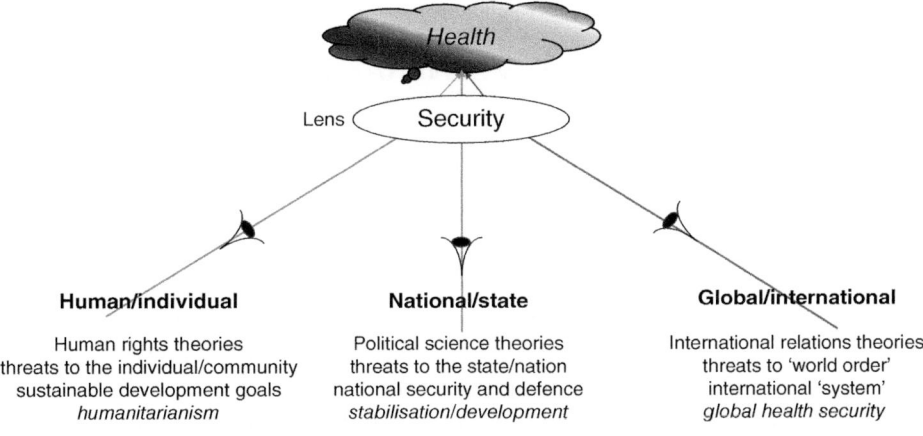

FIGURE 16.1 Perspectives on health and security.

the Sphere Handbook. It first looked at the response of a whole health system to a crisis including the international humanitarian system. It then considered the care of physical trauma patients and the concept of a chain or pathway of care. Next was a review of the impact of war on communicable disease, and the link to the concept of GHS. The last two chapters on physical disease described the impact of war on maternal and child health services and on care for non-communicable disease and palliative care. The final chapter in this section examined war and its impact on mental health, both on armed forces personnel and also on civilian populations exposed to war. Part 3 covered two further topics, research into health and insecurity, and policy development for security and health. Each chapter of the book has also provided a learning activity to explore the wider context of each topic and a case study for a particular dimension of the topic. The material presented has been supported by citations to authoritative references and signposting to other sources and resources.

The overall learning outcomes from studying this book are to:

- Set the foundations for a systematic understanding of interdependent concepts from the fields of international relations, security studies, and global health as they relate to the analysis of global health, security, and war
- Familiarise readers with foundational concepts underlying health threats as risks to human, national, and global security
- Explore the role of health sciences and health services in the development of national and supra-national capabilities to protect security, healthcare services and other critical national infrastructures

The reader will have gained the foundational skills to apply this knowledge in the evaluation of the policies, plans, and responses to security and health crises in the future. Unfortunately, at the time of writing, the context for global security and international relations seems more uncertain and with a greater risk of significant conflict between world powers than at any time since the Second World War. The next sections will consider the potential evolution of health impacts of three contemporary security crises.

COVID-19 AS A WARNING OF VULNERABILITY TO FUTURE PANDEMICS

Chapter 2 described how the threat of a pandemic was forecast as a high-impact/high-likelihood risk in many security risk assessments. Previous public health emergencies of international concern (PHEICs) had generated considerable discussion about GHS and measures to detect and manage a potential outbreak. The COVID-19 pandemic demonstrated the lack of capability and capacity of governments to respond. Overall, there is evidence that higher GHS index scores were associated with lower excess comparative mortality ratios (CMRs) during the COVID-19 pandemic. Perversely, within this positive message, some individual countries that had scored highly on the GHS index were not so highly ranked when listed by CMR. This variation seemed to be most strongly correlated with government effectiveness [1]. It is also notable that the Module 1 report of the UK COVID-19 inquiry observed that the United Kingdom was widely considered to be one of the best-prepared countries to respond to a pandemic before the COVID-19 crisis. Yet the actual performance of politicians and government demonstrated strategic flaws in the assessment of risks and the management of civil emergencies [2].

In May 2020, on behalf of the World Health Assembly, the Director General of the World Health Organization (WHO) convened an Independent Panel for Pandemic Preparedness and Response to make recommendations to curb the COVID-19 pandemic and to advise how to respond to any future outbreak of infectious disease to ensure it would not become another catastrophic pandemic.[1] The first report was submitted to the World Health Assembly in May 2021. The most recent follow-on report published in June 2024 described a 'dangerous lack of progress' against the 2021 recommendations. This was considered in the case study in Chapter 15.

Inevitably, the COVID-19 pandemic increased the focus on health and biosecurity within national security strategies in order to mitigate the risks of catastrophic outcomes from health threats. A reader of this book may wish to consider how this focus might shift or diminish in the future if other sources of strategic threat become more prominent topics in the debates over national and international security. It is concerning that many countries' health systems have not yet cleared the serious backlog of clinical referrals that were deferred during the COVID-19 crisis. Urgent and emergency care is also under severe stress because the social care system for caring for elderly patients is not able to demand for discharge care after hospital admission. This poses a substantial risk of lack of capacity to absorb a surge of demand from another health crisis.

WAR AS DESTRUCTION: UKRAINE

The international community had been appalled by the military tactics and the human consequences of the conduct of war by the Assad regime and their Russian allies during the Syrian civil war in the second decade of the 21st century. The Russian annexation of the Donbas and Crimea regions of Ukraine in 2014 was a strategic shock. It had been hoped that the second Minsk Agreement of 2015 would have been sufficient to stabilise the conflict. However, Russia attempted a full-scale invasion of Ukraine in February 2022. Although the Ukrainian defence prevented the seizure of Kiev and the collapse of the Ukrainian government, some 20% of Eastern Ukrainian territory had been captured. This created the most intense war and the largest refugee crisis in Europe since the Second World War.

This war is being conducted using the most modern multi-domain military equipment. The intensity and sophistication of air defences have restricted the use of helicopters and aircraft close to the front line. However, both types of aircraft have been used to launch stand-off bombs and missiles to attack the frontlines and deeper targets. The land battle has seen the return of trench warfare and urban warfare. Artillery and missile bombardment have been as intense as the Second World War. Although armoured vehicles offer some protection, this war has seen the absolute domination of low-cost drones for reconnaissance, precision dropping of low-payload bombs, and first-person view (FPV) suicide drones. The war is also being fought in the electromagnetic spectrum to disrupt communications, especially control of drones. The Ukrainian forces have been especially effective at using drones in the Black Sea to disrupt Russian naval forces. It is also being fought in the cyber-domain and information domains both within Ukraine and more widely. Russian 'cyber-criminals' have caused significant disruption to health information services in the United Kingdom and have also attacked other countries.

Both sides have suffered substantial military deaths though the exact figures are closely guarded secrets. In an unprecedented post on Twitter (X) on 8 December 2024, President Zelinsky announced that Ukraine had lost 43,000 soldiers killed with 370,000 cases of medical assistance for the wounded.[2] Although he suggested that Ukrainian data showed approximately half of the soldiers wounded in action are later returning to the battlefield, it means that 185,000 military personnel are unfit for further action. President Zelinsky compared the Ukrainian numbers with an estimate of Russian losses of 198,000 killed and more than 550,000 wounded. Conscription is drawing a large proportion of the youth generation into the armed forces though this is increasingly unpopular. A significant number of Ukrainian civilians have been killed or wounded, and there continues to be a substantial internal and international displacement of Ukrainian women and children. The secondary and tertiary impacts of the war are having severe effects on access and quality of general health services for the Ukrainian population [3].

The war has also been characterised by a disregard towards International Humanitarian Law. There is clear evidence of direct targeting and damage to hospitals and medical transports. The Russian campaign has deliberately targeted civilian infrastructure including national power and key dams. There is evidence of mass deportation of civilians and abduction of children. Prisoners have been tortured and summarily executed. There are also allegations of Russian tactical use of unknown gases.

The war in Ukraine is an indication of the character of a contemporary war involving two equally equipped armed forces. The intensity of front-line battles reflects the destructive power of modern weapons. Although the explosive power of missiles and artillery is unchanged, the drone has transformed the lethality of short-range combat. The Russian approach to the conduct of war seems unchanged since the Second World War with the outcome on the battlefield the only measure of success and a disregard to the limitations of war under International Humanitarian Law. There is a palpable sense of foreboding amongst countries lying on the border with Russia and a more intense focus on balancing this with improved military capability amongst NATO countries.

INTRACTIBLE CONFLICT AND HEALTH: THE FIGHT FOR ISRAELI AND PALESTINIAN IDENTITY

The abhorrent attacks by members of the Palestinian group Hamas on the territory of Israel on 7 October 2023 set off a new wave of instability and violence in the endemic conflict between Israel, Palestinians and wider regional adversaries. In addition to causing a catastrophic loss of life and a massive number of war injured, the Israeli military campaign has destroyed or damaged a very significant proportion of the civilian infrastructure in Gaza. The violence has also extended to the Palestinian West Bank and the Israel–Lebanon border, threatened international maritime trade through the Suez Canal, and heightened the risk of a sustained war between Israel and Iran. Whilst there has been widespread condemnation of the Hamas attack, there is also increasing criticism of Israeli strategy and tactics in the campaign in Gaza with suggestions of multiple transgressions of International Humanitarian Law in regard to the use of siege of civilians as a tactic, targeting and collateral killing of civilians, restriction of access to medical care, and inhumane treatment of prisoners. The regional political situation has been further complicated by the collapse of the Assad regime in Syria and the emergence of a government under the Hay'at Tahrir al-Sham (HTS) group which has been previously sanctioned as an Islamist paramilitary organisation.

The Syrian civil war had catastrophic consequences for Syrians with local and regional migration causing significant challenges for host countries. The dramatic increase in violence has already had devastating consequences for the health of Palestinians in Gaza. There have also been significant numbers of killed and wounded in the other areas of conflict. This war, conflict, and confrontation have the potential to cause more harm to more people in the Middle East than any of the previous Arab–Israeli wars. In spite of this, the global effort to emphasise International Humanitarian Law seems to have been unheeded by the armed actors [4].

IS CONTEMPORARY WAR MORE INHUMANE?

The wars in Ukraine and the Middle East are a reminder of the destructive power of modern weapons. The modern drone as a low-cost, loitering means of surveillance and attack has made the battlefield more transparent. The impact of war on civilians remains unchanged. If they can move, they become internally displaced and refugees. If they cannot move due to siege, they are deprived of water, food, shelter, sanitation, and access to healthcare. The impact of these wars on communities and societies will be felt across generations.

The aggressors in both regional conflicts intend to destroy the will and capacity of their enemies to fight through destruction and attrition. It could be argued that the actual strategic conduct of these wars is not different to the conduct of previous wars fought by these aggressors. The only redeeming factor is that weapons of mass destruction have not been used, except for the tactical use of incapacitant gases. Unfortunately, it would seem that war will always be inhumane and catastrophic, and directed by rational people even if their motivation is inhumane. With this inevitability in mind, it remains equally important to understand the reasons for war, to champion International Humanitarian Law, to document the impact of war on health, to continually improve the management of health conditions arising from war, and to advocate for policies to minimise the likelihood of war and other humanitarian emergencies.

WORKING IN HEALTH, SECURITY, AND CONFLICT

Many readers of this book may consider working in the fields of health, security, and conflict. This section considers how to determine the education, training, and experience that might be desirable to work in this sector plus the types of employment available. The first consideration is motivation and appetite for risk. This book describes the impact of humanitarian emergencies and conflict on health, including the need to mobilise organisations, people, and resources to mitigate this. Chapter 8 explained that most of the practical responses will be local or regional; however, international organisations and supportive national governments are part of the response. Many people working in this sector have a powerful altruistic desire to try to improve the lives and well-being of affected populations. Most organisations are actively trying to 'decolonise' the humanitarian workforce by employing local or regional personnel and ensuring equity across race and gender. Thus, entry-level roles for international staff can be limited and tend to be as volunteers or interns paid a stipend. Substantive roles are adequately paid by Western standards but are often on time-limited contracts with substantial job insecurity. Permanent employment tends to be for more senior appointments and is dependent on extensive field experience. All field roles will require substantial time away from home countries (but may come with a rest and recuperation (R&R) package). Chapter 14 described some of the risks associated with fieldwork. Volunteers or employees should do their own 'due diligence' to check that their appetite for personal risk at least matches the expectations of their organisation and that they are covered by a credible health and repatriation insurance policy. Most humanitarian and government organisations will require field workers to undertake some form of hostile environment training and to comply with their protection policies.

Many workers in the health field will have a primary qualification as a health professional (doctor, nurse, psychologist, public health) with post-graduate clinical experience. A master's degree in public health, global health, tropical medicine, or development would often be expected for work in a humanitarian or development field. There are also a variety of free online courses in a wide range of humanitarian or development topics. These may provide certificates that would demonstrate an interest in the field (examples are listed at the end of the chapter). An alternative route would be education in international relations, politics, or development with a view to generalist roles in management or leadership. Entry-level roles in this stream are also likely to be as volunteers or interns in headquarters or national organisations prior to international employment. It is also possible to get into this field by government employment in the diplomatic service, development agencies, or the armed forces. A start point is to look at the profiles of jobs within the sector posted on organisation's websites. The jobs section of ReliefWeb (https://reliefweb.int/jobs) is a global broker of humanitarian and development jobs. This source provides an indication of the types and names of organisations working in the field and the profiles of relevant jobs. It is also worthwhile to attend conferences and seminars on humanitarian topics to chat with current practitioners.

FINAL CONCLUSION

Well done for reaching the end of this book 😊. We hope that you have enjoyed its contents and that you have learned something about the relationships between health, security, and war. If you wish to learn more, you might consider undertaking formal education at the master's level in the topic. You might also consider taking some free online courses on humanitarian and disaster topics that are available from the following sources:

Kaya – https://kayaconnect.org/
FutureLearn – https://www.futurelearn.com/ – search for 'humanitarian'
Disaster Ready – https://www.disasterready.org/
Martin Bricknell
Richard Sullivan

NOTES

1. The reports of the Independent Panel for Pandemic Preparedness and Response are at https://theindependentpanel.org/.
2. President Zelinsky [@ZelenskyyUa]. (8 December 2024) 'Yesterday, I visited President @EmmanuelMacron at the Élysée Palace and had a good meeting with President @realDonaldTrump.' [Post]. X. https://x.com/ZelenskyyUa/status/1865709519352873408.

REFERENCES

1. Ledesma, J.R., Isaac, C.R., Dowell, S.F. et al. (2023). Evaluation of the Global Health Security Index as a predictor of COVID-19 excess mortality standardised for under-reporting and age structure. *BMJ Global Health* 8 (7): e012203. https://doi.org/10.1136/bmjgh-2023-012203.
2. UK COVID-19 Inquiry (2024). *Module 1: The Resilience and Preparedness of the United Kingdom*. London: Stationary Office. https://covid19.public-inquiry.uk/documents/module-1-full-report/ (accessed 4 March 2025).
3. Haque, U., Bukhari, M.H., Fiedler, N. et al. (2024). A comparison of Ukrainian hospital services and functions before and during the Russia-Ukraine war. *JAMA Health Forum.* 5 (5): e240901. https://doi.org/10.1001/jamahealthforum.2024.0901.
4. Gostin, L.O. and Goodwin, M.B. (2024). Wars in Gaza and beyond: why protecting the sacredness of health matters. *JAMA* 331 (3): 191–192. https://doi.org/10.1001/jama.2023.26391.

Index

Page number followed by 'f' refers to figures. Page numbers followed by 't' refer to tables. Page number followed by 'n' refers to notes.

Handbook of Global Health, Security, and War, First Edition. Edited by Martin Bricknell and Richard Sullivan.
© 2025 John Wiley & Sons Ltd. Published 2025 by John Wiley & Sons Ltd.

Printed and bound by CPI Group (UK) Ltd, Croydon, CR0 4YY

19/08/2025

14720489-0001